Allergy Made Simple

AF880497

Allergy Made Simple

For those who are allergic *and* for those who might become so

2nd revised and expanded edition

Rüdiger Wahl, PhD
Hamburg, Germany

With 8 tables and 30 drawings,
including 21 cartoons by Sandra Wahl, Hamburg, Germany
Forewords by Prof. A. Kaplan, MD, Prof. A.L. de Weck, MD,
and Prof. K. Ch. Bergmann MD

Hogrefe & Huber Publishers
Seattle · Toronto · Göttingen · Bern

Library of Congress Cataloging-in-Publication Data
Library of Congress Cataloging-in-Publication Data is available via the
Library of Congress Marc Database under the
LC Catalog Card Number 2002101956

National Library of Canada Cataloguing in Publication Data

Wahl, Rüdiger
Allergy made simple : for those who are allergic and for those who might become so
2nd rev. and expanded ed.
Translation of: Allergie ganz einfach
ISBN 0-88937-254-3

1. Allergy – Popular works. I. Title
RC 584.W313 2002 616.97 C2002-900870-0

ISBN 0-88937-254-3

Hogrefe & Huber Publishers, Seattle · Toronto · Bern · Göttingen
© 2002 by Hogrefe & Huber Publishers

USA: P.O. Box 2487, Kirkland, WA 98083-2487, Phone (425) 820-1500, Fax (425) 823-8324, E-mail hh@hhpub.com
CANADA: 12 Bruce Park Avenue, Toronto, Ontario M4P 2S3, Phone (416) 482-6339, E-mail hh@hhpub.com
SWITZERLAND: Länggass-Strasse 76, CH-3000 Bern 9 Phone (031) 300-4500, Fax (031) 300-4590
GERMANY: Rohnsweg 25, D-37085 Göttingen, Phone (0551) 496090, Fax (0551) 4960988, E-mail hhpub@hogrefe.de

No part of this book may be reproduced, stored in a retrieval system, or transmitted, in any form or by any means, electronic, mechanical, photocopying, microfilming, recording or otherwise, without the written permission of the publisher.

Printed in Germany

Foreword to the second expanded English edition

Allergy Made Simple, by Rüdiger Wahl, is a unique book which summarizes the most up-to-date information regarding the causes of "allergy" and its prevention and treatment, employing a practical, readable, and thoroughly enjoyable approach.

It is written primarily for patients who suffer from allergic diseases. However, anyone with an interest in allergic diseases will find material in it that is of interest and informative. The book surveys the many substances that cause allergic symptoms and discusses the symptoms that can arise, approaches to distinguish which allergen is responsible for symptoms such as rhinitis, asthma, dermatitis, and urticaria, and available treatments.

Dr. Wahl has been updating the information on a regular basis, thus the current rendition represents the second English (and the fifth German) edition incorporating new information such as the possible use of cloned allergens for diagnostic and therapeutic purposes. It also updates our knowledge of cross-reacting allergenic determinants, that is, how allergy to one substance can lead to symptoms when exposed to a seemingly very different substance.

One of the most striking features of the book is the liberal use of photographs, humorous cartoons to emphasize a particular point, and even songs to lighten the spirit. Practical hints are offered throughout.

Dr. Wahl's contribution is an important addition to the available literature for patients with allergy, and I can recommend it wholeheartedly.

Spring 2002

Professor Allen Kaplan, MD
President, World Allergy Organization
Division of Pulmonary Allergy and Critical Care
Medical University of South Carolina, Charleston, SC

Foreword to the first English edition

Allergy Made Simple is in many ways an unusual book. The author. Rüdiger Wahl, is basically a laboratory man, who went on from being a young PhD student analyzing allergen extracts in the corner of a secluded industrial laboratory to become a well known scientist with a mastery of many facets of allergology, including very practical and even exotic clinical observations. In a way, the cold extract has gone back to where it came from, a blossoming and multicolored flower!

Most introductory books on allergy written by medical doctors read rather like (over)simplified academic treatises, which usually bore non-specialist readers with strange names and difficult concepts (have you ever heard of "pathophysiology"?). This book is written by somebody who not only understands allergens and the numerous causes of allergies, the sources of all that sneezing, coughing, and itching, but can also explain them – clearly, and with wit and humor as well. It reads like a walk through the botanical garden of life, as a wretched allergic patient experiences it. In so doing, Rüdiger Wahl emphasizes many unexpected links and encounters (called "cross-reactions"), enabling the attentive reader to avoid them in the future.

Indeed, beyond describing all that can be done for them in terms of diagnosis and therapy, this book teaches patients how to "live with allergy," which is far more important for coping with allergy than any doctor. In this sense, *Allergy Made Simple* is most valuable, and can be recommended to anyone who knows or believes themselves to be allergic.

The book is also a quite remarkable demonstration of how one can talk or write about serious or itchy matters with some humor and a light spirit, or even sing about them (a collection of allergic pop hits is included here!). It is better to laugh than to sneeze, the author tells us; this is indeed already a form of anti-allergic therapy. I shall recommend this book to all my patients, for sure.

February 1996 — Prof. A. L. de Weck, MD

Foreword to the third German edition

What choice do you have when a tall author – someone whom you can only look up to – asks you to pen a forword to a very charming little book? Of course you immediately accept, and are then faced with the problem of how to praise the work but avoid making the author feel even taller.

I can say with pleasure that I can highly recommend and greatly appreciate *Allergy Made Simple*, for it is a book which makes a pleasant change from so many other writings addressed to allergy patients. There is no book that is quite so delightful and encouraging, that solicits as many chuckles as the one recommended here. I must admit that I have long since made slides from it, without even asking Rüdiger Wahl's permission, and everybody's favorite is the cat, merrily taking a shower.

This impressive and very readable book, now appearing in its third edition, provides allergy patients with the most important points about their illness, its causes, diagnosis, prevention, and therapy. Medical facts are rarely presented in such a cheerful way, and the text clearly illuminates the author's commitment.

I hope this book enjoys many more editions and reaches a wide readership – many thanks to the author.

August 1995 Professor K. Ch. Bergmann, MD

Preface to the fifth German edition

Fortunately, the interest in my little yellow book continues, so that 7 years after the appearance of the first edition, this, the 5th, edition has now become necessary. My goal here too was to bring the book up to date, for example, by adding a section on the city/country phenomenon in allergic illnesses and comments on a newly discovered hidden allergen in food (not revealed here, take a look in the text) – a very interesting fact indeed.

One thing was absolutely necessary: A new illustration (Figure 17) by my niece.

I hope my readers continue to enjoy my little book and have a few "aha" experiences to boot.

Let me repeat what Professor U. Wahn (Berlin, Germany) mentioned in his book review in *Allergo Journal* (Volume 322, 1999, p. 7): "I recommend this book to be best enjoyed at the end of the day with a glass of red wine in the other hand." What can I say: Cheers!

October 2000 Rüdiger Wahl

Preface to the fourth German edition

Why so quickly a fourth edition? After many reprints, the third edition is presently out of print, and it seemed logical to use the opportunity of a new edition to make some changes and add some things, in part to reflect the comments of my readers and in part to bring the material up to date. Since the appearance of the 3rd edition much has happened in the area of allergy research. For example, genetically modified (recombinant) allergens have now been implemented in studies concerning *in vivo* and *in vitro* allergy diagnostics. Initial studies have also been made on the use of protein particles (peptides) in immunotherapy. Individual allergens have been described down to their basic amino acids. This is all very interesting, though strictly not the theme of this volume, being much too detailed and limited. Rather, it was my desire to revise, change, improve and expand some of the information given here. Among other things the table dealing with allergen cross-reactivity needed to be updated and restructured, since our knowledge concerning cross-reactivity is, in my opinion, very important for both the allergic patient and the treating physician. Further, another important area of allergy needed to be discussed: animal allergy. As with humans, allergies in animals are also clearly on the increase, and I wanted to provide some further information for the readers. One thing, however, remains, I would hope: that the text and illustrations of the 4th edition still provide the reader with pleasure. My niece has contributed three new illustrations.

June 1998 Rüdiger Wahl

Preface to the third German edition

Why a revised edition after only 18 months? Happily for me, the first and second edition of my book enjoyed great success with allergy sufferers and non-sufferers alike, including doctors and professors. TV and radio stations, magazines, and health insurance companies all took notice of my little yellow book, treating it very positively. I received many helpful hints toward making it even more "worthwhile." In the last year in particular there have been several new theories as to why the number of allergy sufferers is increasing. So, to share all of this, here is the revised edition, written, like the first one, under sunny skies – this time in Greece. Its aim is not only to provide a clear discussion of allergies but perhaps to reduce some of the fears people have of them. Amidst the suffering, try to keep in mind that pollen allows nature to blossom and bloom, producing a colorful and beautiful world, not just one which makes our eyes stream and noses run.

I hope you have fun browsing through my third edition.

June 1995 Rüdiger Wahl

Preface to the first German edition

This little book doesn't claim to be highly scientific. For scientists there are already many better and more comprehensive books discussing allergic disorders from a rigorous medical and scientific viewpoint. But this book is not intended just for scientists and doctors (although I'd be very happy if they all read it). It is meant to entertain both those who suffer from allergies and those who don't, providing information about allergic disorders which may in themselves be of interest. Although allergies are very serious and the allergic endure a great deal of suffering, this small book is intended to raise a little smile.

Enjoy!

August 1993 Rüdiger Wahl

Contents

Things you should know

Acaricides:	A substance or preparation for killing acarids (mites and ticks) (spray or foam)
ÄDA	Allergy Congress held in Bonn, Germany, in September 2000. A number of lectures held at this wonderful allergy congress inspired many changes introduced in this edition.
Airborne pollen:	See p. 28
Allergens:	Substances which can cause allergic reactions such as pollen, house dust mites, food, drugs, etc.
Allergic people	See p. 61
Alster	A river in Hamburg, Germany, along the edges of which I sat and corrected much of the 4th edition. The sun was shining.
Allergologist:	Specialist for allergic disorders.
American Academy of Allergy, Asthma and Immunology:	Thank you for your support by sending me material about allergies in the USA.
Anamnesis:	The medical history of a patient as recorded by the physician to reveal, among other things, any allergic reactions present.
Anaphylactic shock:	Serious allergic reaction combined with circulatory collapse. A physician must be called immediately.
Antihistamine drug:	Medication which works by blocking the cells' receptors for histamine (see p. 106).
Antibodies:	Proteins which act on (i. e., chemically react with) specific antigens (allergens). IgG, IgA, IgM, IgE, and IgD all have different structures and functions (see p. 107).
Asthma and Allergy Foundation:	Thank you for the information material about allergy in the USA.
Asthma bronchiale:	Reversible constriction of the respirato-

	ry tract, shortness of breath, wheezing noises.
Atkinson, Dr. P.:	Thank you for your support. – Allergy in the UK.
Atopy:	Inherited allergic predisposition.
Bircher, Dr. A.J.:	Many thanks for the good work together on *Ficus benjamina* allergy.
Bossert, Dr. J.:	My heartfelt thanks for all the proofreading, helpful hints, and an allergologist's professional advice on the three editions.
BPI:	My speeches as part of the lecturing service sponsored by the German Federal Association of Pharmaceutical Industries formed the foundation for the first edition.
Bronchial asthma:	Progressive contraction of the air passages, difficulty breathing, whistling breathing sounds.
Burghardt, B., Wallrafen, A:	My thanks to the staff from the German Association of Allergy and Asthma Sufferers (Deutscher Allergiker- und Asthmatikerbund), Mönchengladbach, for their support and valuable conversations.
Carsten:	It was great being able to work in your music studio – Thanks!
Case history:	Information about an illness (here, allergies) collected by a doctor.
Colleagues:	I thank many colleagues for their excellent and successful, always highly motivated, conscientious collaboration.
Conjunctivitis:	Inflammation of the mucous membrane connected with red, watering, swollen eyes.
Cortisone:	Adrenocortical hormone which has a general anti-inflammatory effect. Should not be used over a long period of time without consulting a physician.
Cross-reactivity:	Various substances contain the same allergenic components.

Debelic, Dr. M.:	It was a great pleasure writing the *in vitro* article for the *Manuale allergologicum* together with you. Thank you for your always interesting professional support.
De Weck, Prof. Dr. A	My thanks for all of the personal and professional discussions.
Desensitization:	Causal therapy to reduce the allergic over-sensitivity of the organism toward allergens; can consist of subcutaneous injections, oral or sublingual application (administration) of allergen extracts such as house dust mites, pollen, etc.
Dermatitis:	Inflammation of the skin
Dimbleby, R.	Thanks for conscientious proofreading and for deciding to have the German edition translated into English.
Early reaction type:	Allergic reactions mediated by IgE (see p. 107).
Eckardt, H.P. and colleagues of Dustri Publishers:	Thanks so very much for your support on the German book, from beginning to end.
Ehl, Dr. W.:	Many thanks for your warm cooperation in editing case studies.
EAST (Enzyme-Allergosorbent Test):	Like RAST, only an enzyme-labeled anti-human IgE is substituted for a radioactively labeled anti-IgE.
Eczema:	Itchy skin disease, redness, weeping, swelling.
Faclam-Wolf, A.:	My thanks to MCA Musikverlag Hamburg for your support (see pp. 24, 28, 61).
Fuerteventura:	There, under the Spanish sun, I wrote most of the first book and proofread the third edition (Feb. '95).
Fuchs, Prof. Dr. E.	Thank you for the many enjoyable discussions both personal and professional.
Fuchs, Dr. Th.:	My thanks for your continuing help in editing case studies, particularly those on latex allergies.

Hamburg, the winter of 1998, which was more like Spring:	Many of the new ideas implemented in the previous edition were hatched while sitting on a yellow leather couch, in the evening and on weekends. Which just goes to show it doesn't have to be Fuerteventura or the southern coast of Crete.
Hauck, P., Oliver, J. and Manassa, D.:	Many thanks to the experts and friends from Port Washington, N.Y.C. Thank you Jerry for your help and proofreading.
Hellerman, M.:	My thanks for your wonderful help in creating the article on neurodermatitis.
Herold, Dr. D.:	My thanks for your warm co-operation in editing case studies.
Histamine:	In allergic reactions, histamine is released from the mast cells and is responsible for the allergic symptoms. It's a so-called mediator substance, also known as a biologically active substance. It's also used as a positive test solution in skin tests.
Hogrefe, Dr. Christine:	My thanks for deciding to have the German edition translated into English.
Hypoallergenic foods:	Foods with an extremely low allergenicity residue, specially suited for allergy sufferers.
Hyposensitization:	See Desensitization
Immunoglobulin E (IgE):	Antibodies which play a decisive role in type 1 allergic reactions (immediate type), first discovered by Johansson and Ishizaka in 1967.
Immunoglobulin G (IgG):	Antibodies which are often strongly increased through hyposensitization. They are intended to protect against the allergen.
Immune therapy:	See Desensitization
Inhaled allergens:	Allergens such as pollen, mold, flour dust etc.
Intracutaneous:	Into the skin
Intracutaneous test:	Allergy test carried out on a patient's back by injecting allergen extracts direct-

ly into the skin, more painful than the skin prick test but at least 1000 times more sensitive.

In vivo: Within a living body

In vitro: In a test-tube, i. e., outside a living body.

Irene: My heartfelt thanks to my beloved wife!

Jorde, Dr. W.: I appreciate so much that I am always able to tap your broad experience concerning allergic illnesses, particularly regarding mold allergy.

Kleinhans, Prof. Dr. D.: My thanks for your wonderful cooperation in clarifying the "gummybear allergy".

Kroidl, Dr. R.: My thanks for your warm cooperation in editing case studies.

Masuch, Prof. Dr. G.: It was highly interesting for me to be able to carry out the study on the influence of ozone on the allergenic activity of pollen.

Müsken, Dr. H.: My thanks for the years of warm cooperation in editing case studies.

Neurodermatitis: Itchy skin irritation

Placebo: A tablet, for example, without an active ingredient and therefore not technically a drug.

Pollen: Male germ cell of a plant, the allergen which causes hay fever, etc.

Pollinosis: Hay fever, caused by pollen

Protein: Allergens are 90–95% proteins or glycoproteins, i. e., proteins with carbohydrates (sugar).

Provocation test: The affected organ is provoked by the suspicious allergen; subdivisions include oral, nasal, conjunctival and bronchial provocation. Particularly important for acquiring an expert opinion concerning occupational diseases.

Pseudo-allergy: Symptomatic reaction which is not allergic: often an intolerance, usually caused by medication.

RAST (Radio-Allergo-Sorbent Test):	*In vitro* test to determine specific IgE serum of a patient; the patient's own serum is used.
Rumball, James and Rachel Kretz	My heartfelt thanks for your warm cooperation and fine translation into English.
Rhinitis:	Cold in the head
Sabine:	Thanks for proofreading the 3rd edition and for your many helpful remarks.
Schultze-Werninghaus, Prof. Dr. G.:	Many thanks for your friendly support of various projects.
Sensitization:	Reaction of the body to allergy-causing substances, caused by frequent contact and characterized by the production of antibodies.
Serum:	Extracted from the blood through centrifugation: 6 ml of blood produce approx. 2–3 ml of serum. *In vitro* tests such as RAST or EAST are carried out with the serum, which is the liquid ingredient in blood plasma.
Skin prick test:	Painless allergy test which consists of introducing the allergen extract into the skin.
Southeast Crete:	It was there at 12.10 pm on the night of June 3, 1994, that I received the inspiration for revising "Allergy Made Simple." As I tossed and turned, unable to sleep, I was kissed by the Greek muse of allergies. I really like such kisses – although I enjoy certain others even more.
Sprung, Dipl.-Doc. V.:	My heartfelt thanks for your very conscientious proofreading of the 5th German edition and your very helpful remarks from the vantage point of an allergy newcomer. Muchas gracias. Keep on running, but stop jogging in the dark. Remember 1712.
Staff:	Many thanks to the staff for their wonderful, always dedicated cooperation.
Subcutaneous:	Under one's skin, i.e., "Darling, you've

	become really subcutaneous," as the song goes.
Sublingual:	Under the tongue.
The Flight of the Pollen:	See page 28
The lonely scientist	See p. 24
Urticaria:	Rash with formation of wheals.
Various German and international scientists, doctors, and friends:	My thanks for your warm and effective cooperation.
Wahl, Dr. G.	Many thanks for helpful comments from a brother and a cardiologist.
Weber, Dr. M.:	Thank you for proofreading the Polish translation of the 4th edition and for your many important remarks from a medical, allergological viewpoint.
Willgeroth, Dr. Th.:	It was fascinating working with you on the relatively seldom sperm allergy. I hope it benefits the woman in question.
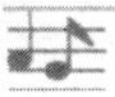	Indicates an anecdote or report on the latest scientific studies.

Where does the word "allergy" come from and what does it actually mean?

The word "allergy"is derived from the Greek "allon argon," which expresses a willingness to react differently, to deviate from the norm. This means that allergic people respond differently to certain substances than non-allergic people do, developing a hypersensitivity leading to illness. Over 40,000 such substances, to which new ones are added every day, can cause hypersensitivity, i. e., allergic reactions in people with a corresponding predisposition.

Are allergies an illness of our times?

Allergies are not confined just to our times; they have been around for hundreds of years. As early as 1570 a man was reported to be allergic to cat hair when, upon entering a room in which a cat had hidden itself, he became agitated, broke out in a sweat and developed blisters on his skin. Allergies have multiplied in recent years, however, and as a result of today's improved knowledge, many hitherto unexplained pathological reactions to certain substances have been diagnosed as allergic.

Scientists estimate, for example, that up to 25–30% of the population in industrialized countries suffer from allergies, and that 41 million Americans have asthma and allergies. They have pinpointed a sharp increase in job-related allergies caused by "occupational materials."

In the United States, 22.4 million people have hay fever (seasonal allergic rhinitis), 10 million have asthma, and 11.8 million are affected by the following allergic conditions: eczema, urticaria (hives), angioedeme (swelling), allergic reaction to food, medication and insect stings. There are three million asthmatics under the age of 18. Seven percent of all US children have asthma. It is the most common cause of pediatric admission to most children's hospitals. Four to five billion dollars are spent each year by those Americans suffering from asthma and allergic disease. In the UK, 20% to 40% of the population suffer from allergies, depending on the source quoted. About 5% of allergic people suffer from atopic dermatitis. Atopic people (see p. 54) primarily suffer from such allergies, but non-atopic people in frequent contact with aggressive-enough substances can also become sensitized and develop allergic reactions as well.

A hairdresser broke out in a rash while giving customers a henna rinse. Serum studies and skin tests (see p. 84) with various henna preparations indicated that the patient had sensitized herself through exposure and had developed an allergic reaction to henna. Red and black henna caused slightly more irritation than the colorless variety. Other substances in a hairdressing salon such as hydrogen peroxide, used for dying hair blonde, can cause allergic reactions as well.

A goldsmith who, in the course of his work, had to use spindle tree shavings in treating the gold, showed an allergic reaction to the shavings. After avoiding them for several months, the allergic reaction disappeared.

As occurrences of such job-related skin diseases increased in Germany (to take one country as an example) by 84% between 1978 and 1989, the list of job-related allergies could just go on and on.

Can allergies indirectly cause death in non-allergic people?

A curious story with a simple enough explanation: King Richard III of England is said to have been allergic to strawberries. After eating some of the fruit he developed a swelling, a rash, and diarrhea, all typical symptoms of a food allergy. Since the word "allergy" at that time did not exist, he suspected his food had been poisoned, and had one of his servants beheaded. As you can see, life has (had) its dangers even if you're not allergic. Today we are aware of many food allergies (see pp. 69), and fortunately for the rest of the population only those who are allergic are in any danger!

When were allergies first described?

Hay fever was first clinically described in 1819. It is primarily caused by pollen from grass, grains, trees and herbs. Figure 1 shows various types of pollen as seen under a microscope. Figure 2 is a caricature of pollen attacking a man and his exaggerated but unsuccessful attempts at defending himself.

As pollen is airborne only at specific times of the year, we refer to hay fever as a seasonal allergy, but there are also perennial allergies, in which patients are exposed to allergens such as house dust mites (see p. 18) all year round. People who are allergic only to pollens, therefore, do not suffer for as long as those who are allergic to house dust mites.

What is pollen?

A pollen grain is the male cell necessary for the propagation of seed plants. It is released by one plant and transported by an insect or the wind to pollinate another. Plants pollinated by insects have colorful blossoms and produce just a few, heavy pollen grains that are de-

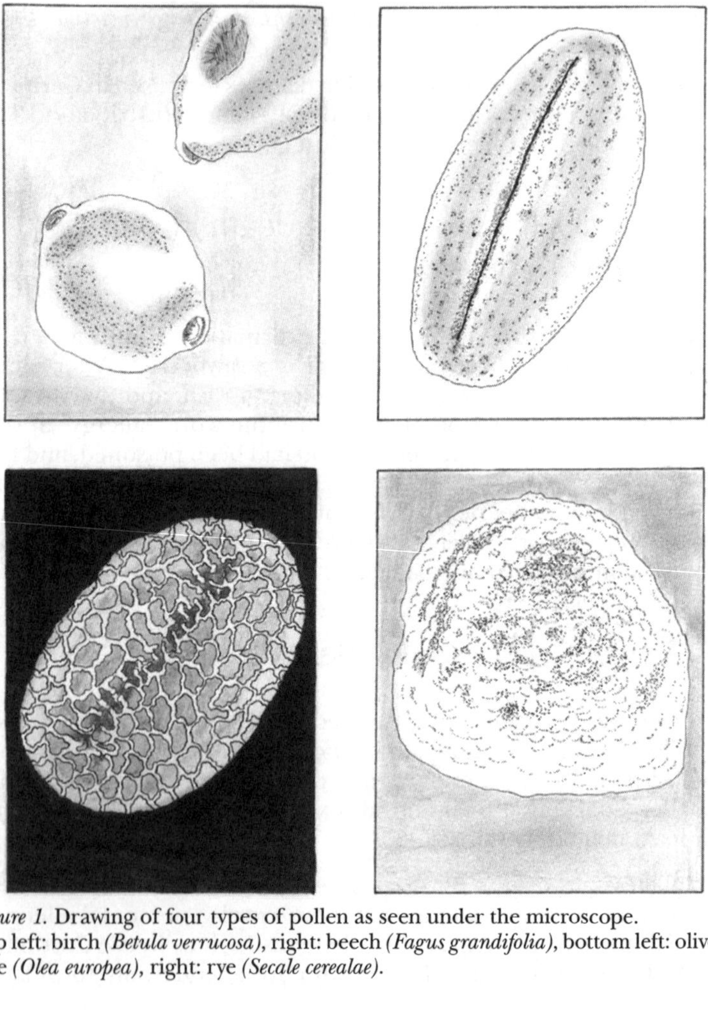

Figure 1. Drawing of four types of pollen as seen under the microscope.
Top left: birch *(Betula verrucosa)*, right: beech *(Fagus grandifolia)*, bottom left: olive tree *(Olea europea)*, right: rye *(Secale cerealae)*.

signed to stick to the insects' legs. Allergic reactions to flowering plants are only possible in people who come in close contact with them, and allergies caused by flowers like chrysanthemums, daisies and begonias occur mostly among gardeners and florists. These flowers pose no great threat to people who suffer from classic pollen allergies. It's not the flowers which cause the real trouble but the green plants, with windblown pollen that is released in enormous amounts into the air. The most important types of pollen in Germany are grass pollen, grain pollen, pollen from trees such as birch, alder, or hazel, and plants like mugwort and plantain.

In the US the pollen of such trees as elm, birch, ash, hickory, poplar, sycamore, maple, cypress, and walnut is often the cause of early spring hay fever. Late spring and early summer hay fever is usually caused by pollinating grasses including timothy, Bermuda, orchard, sweet vernal, red top, and some blue grasses.

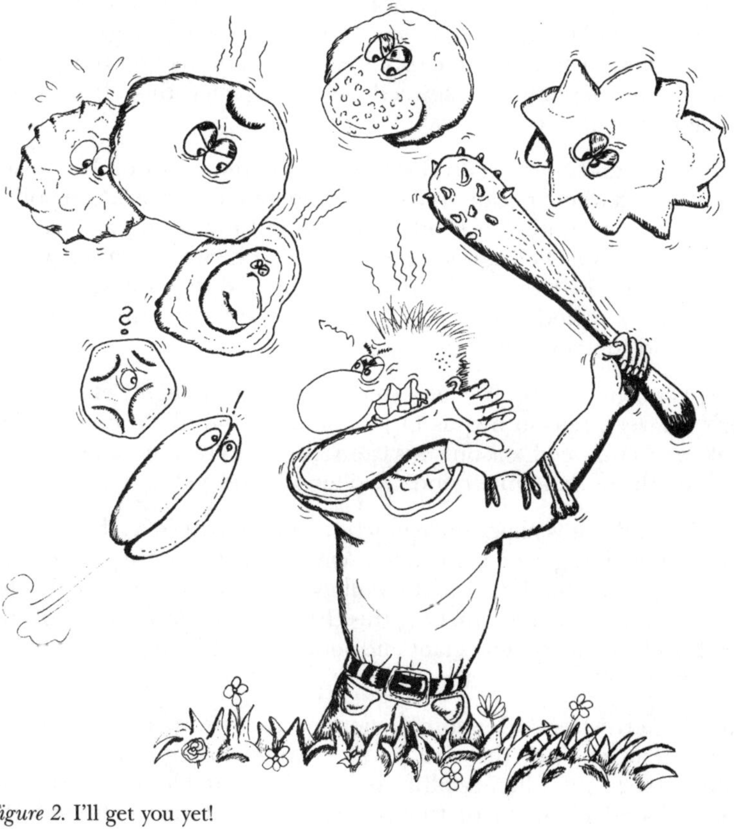

Figure 2. I'll get you yet!

Besides ragweed, which is considered to be the pollen most responsible for seasonal allergic rhinitis in North America, there are other weeds that can cause pollen allergy, including sagebrush, pigweed, tumbleweed, Russian thistle and cockleweed.

Each plant has a period of pollination, which does not vary much from year to year, though weather conditions can effect the amount of pollen in the air at any one time. As the pollinating season occurs later in the year the farther north one goes, obviously hay fever also occurs later in these regions. Trees pollinate earliest, from February or March to April or May, though, this may fluctuate in different locations, starting in April in the Northern United States and varying to as early as January in the South. Grasses follow next in the cycle, beginning pollination in May and continuing until mid-July. Weeds usually pollinate in late summer.

The Eastern states experience three different pollen seasons. Three pollens, particularly oak, sycamore and birch, are prevalent during the months of March through May. In May, June and July, grass pollen is abundant, including orchard, blue grass, timothy and red top. In August and September, ragweed pollen appears, though in lesser quantities than in other areas.

The South and south central states include the states of Tennessee and Georgia where pecans, red cedars and mulberries produce pollen from February until June and Bermuda and Johnson grass are present until frost. The ragweed hay fever season runs from August to late October. In Florida, Texas, Louisiana, and the Gulf area, pollinating trees include pecan, oak, and elm. Grasses include the Bermuda and Johnson varieties.

Florida's southern tip is nearly free of ragweed though Central Florida's ragweed season begins in June and lasts until November. The Gulf area's ragweed season runs from August to November. In Texas, the months of September and October are affected.

The Central states experience much the same pattern as the Eastern states, though ragweed is the major cause of hay fever in this region, with a quarter million tons of pollen blown into the area during August and September, making this the largest concentration of the plant in the country. The giant and short ragweed are the most prevalent here.

The Western states offer some relief because the area produces less pollen than most of the rest of the country due to lower ragweed pollen levels and a higher altitude. However, tumbleweed and sagebrush, found in much of this region, cause adverse reactions for ragweed sufferers, and the tree and grass seasons are similar to those found in the Central states.

The major pollens which cause allergies in the UK are grasses, particularly Timothy grass *(Phleum pratense)*, Cocksfoot *(Dactylis glomerata)*, and ryegrass *(Lolium perenne)*. Tree and weed pollens are of much less significance.

These types of pollen are all transported by the wind. Conifers are also well known pollen producers, but for the most part they are only slightly allergenic, if at all.

How much pollen is contained in an ear of rye or a hazelnut tree?

Since many people are allergic to pollen, there must be a lot of it in the air to keep allergic people "entertained"! There are 4.2 million pollen grains in only one (1) ear of rye, and around 600 million grains in a middle-sized hazelnut tree! If you stop to consider how many ears of rye it takes to make a rye field and how many rye fields there are, you can imagine the amount of rye pollen flying around "polluting" the air!

In central Europe, for instance, this means an average of 27,000 pollen grains for every square centimeter. To be even more facetious, you could go so far as to say that pollen pollutes the environment to a greater extent than car exhaust and industrial plants. I personally, however, far prefer pollen in the air to the stench caused by automobiles and industry in a big city.

Can the allergens in pollen be found everywhere?

As most countries usually have a wide variety of flora, various distinct pollen allergies emerge depending on the country's indigenous plant life. In Germany, for instance, people are allergic to grass and rye; in Scandinavia, to birch; in Italy, Spain and Greece, to olive trees and Parietaria; and in the United States, to ragweed. But people allergic to ragweed can now be found near Frankfurt, Germany due to the US soldiers stationed there, who have unintentionally smuggled seeds into Germany in the cuffs of their pants. In fact ragweed now grows near the airport in Frankfurt. In Japan, Japanese cedar causes grief to those who are allergic to pollen. However, things are not that simple: Even pollen from another country, such as olive tree pollen, can affect people everywhere – even when olive trees don't grow there – if they happen to be allergic to ash and lilac (see p. 65). As you can see, there are regional differences in how various types of pollen cause allergies.

How to be informed if you're allergic to pollen

Like everything else in most parts of the world, the course of airborne pollen is regulated, in this case via radio announcements: "Attention, low-flying grass and rye pollen approaching from the left. If pollen is spotted, signal left, then turn right." Okay, this is an exaggeration, but people who are allergic to pollen receive ample information in order to protect themselves or at least be prepared. But where does the radio station get the information? It comes from the "Pollen information service" which, with the aid of pollen traps, collects data on all the pollen in the air.

What is a pollen trap?

Figure 3 is a very rough sketch. The pollen trap is mounted on a building and consists – in simple terms – of a revolving cylinder covered with a strip of double sided tape which traps the pollen and other particles in the air. When the strip is removed, it is divided into smaller sections and the pollen grains are dyed, making it possible to identify (Fig. 1) and count them under the microscope. After considerable calculation, it is possible to report both the type and the amount of pollen in the air. These pollen traps can also determine and identify the number of mold spores like *Cladosporium herbarum* flying around. As these are known to stick to pollen grains, people allergic to the one should be tested (see pp. 84–92) and if necessary treated (see p. 93) for allergic reactions to the other and vice versa.

What can the allergic driver do?

The only thing that truly relieves stuffed streets and cramped highways is to leave your car at home (something I find very difficult to do). The best remedy for road rage is to smile back, even if it is difficult. And what helps against pollen in the air? Pollen filters like those found in some cars, whether standard or as an extra, is one solution. Such a pollen filter keeps pollen from entering the inside of a car. Sneezing, a runny nose and watery eyes clearly diminish the concentration of any driver. Obviously, for the filters to do their job,

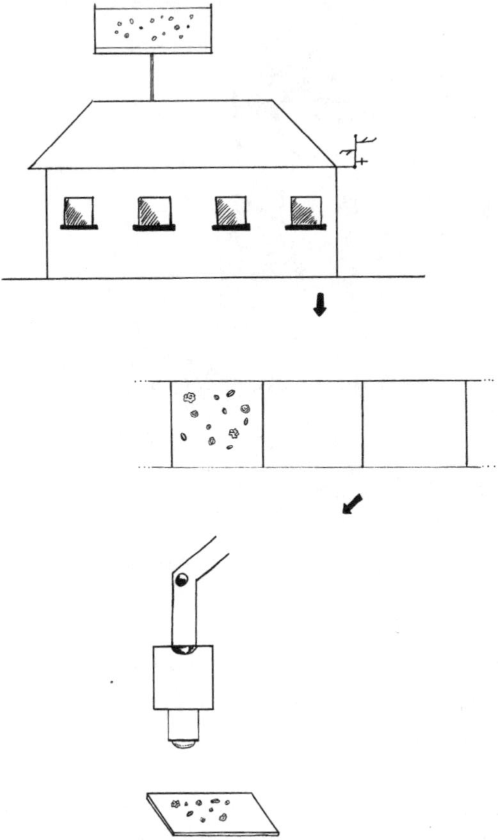

Figure 3. From top to bottom, a simplified representation of a pollen trap: pollen trap attached to the roof, pollen on the strips of tape, pollen identification under the microscope.

all windows and any sliding roof should be kept closed during pollen season. You might consider getting one or having one installed the next time you switch cars.

What further help is available?

Allergy sufferers can avail themselves of so-called pollen calendars, which are classified into those for romantics (Fig. 4) and those for realists (see Appendixes). The pollen calendar provides a clear description of when pollen is airborne and when the levels of a particular pollen are likely to reach "dangerous" levels.

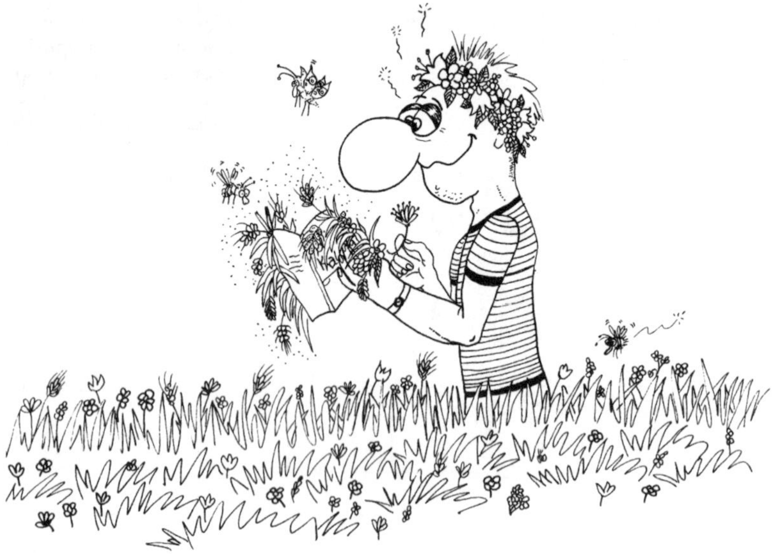

Figure 4. Pollen calendar for romantics, greetings from Constable!

What makes your day if you're allergic to pollen and ruins it if you're in the business of manufacturing allergen extracts?

Rainy days bring relief if you're allergic to pollen because rain causes pollen to drop. Spending the pollen season in Alaska or on Helgoland (a small island in the North Sea off the coast of Germany) will also bring relief as there is almost no airborne pollen there. But why does rain annoy those in the business of manufacturing allergen extracts for therapy? The less people suffer, the less they need therapy (see p. 93), resulting in a fall in the sales of therapeutic preparations. But the next dry spring will surely come, and runny noses will return, creating misery for allergy sufferers and boosting sales for extract manufacturers! This, of course, is what helps me and many other colleagues like me earn a living.

Airborne pollen: The country versus the city

The pollen concentration in the countryside is highest during the day while in the city it peaks in the evenings between 8 and 9 p. m. Allergy sufferers in the city should therefore keep their windows closed particularly in the evenings but also in the mornings. Pollen is released early in the day, carried high into the air around noon and sinks back to earth in the late afternoon, often many miles away. When planning their gardens, people allergic to pollen should make sure not to plant those shrubs to which they are particularly allergic!

Why do people who are allergic to tree pollen suffer in January and May?

Many people allergic to tree pollen in Germany or the UK get allergy symptoms as early as January, sometimes even in December, and then again in May, something they often fail to understand. This is because tree allergies often stem from hazel pollen (December/January) as well as from birch pollen (late April/early May), as these types of pollen are cross-reactive (see p. 64). In other words, they share the same allergens. The warmer the winter, the earlier the hazel trees bloom, causing allergy sufferers grief. Here is yet another reason – from the point of view of allergologists – to actively help conserve the environment and diminish the greenhouse effect, preventing those dreaded warmer temperatures from inducing hazel trees to bloom in October and November!

Similarly, people who are allergic to grass pollen are also allergic to rye pollen, because of their cross-reactivity, and should avoid rye fields during their pollen season at all costs.

Pollen and the environment

Studies with electron microscopes show that chemicals from industrial waste gas, automobile exhaust, and diesel soot attach themselves to many types of pollen. Some scientists speculate that such pollution causes the allergens in the pollen to become more aggressive. While it is probable that allergens from polluted pollen are more efficiently released and more easily penetrate the mucous membrane of the patient's nose, it cannot yet conclusively be said that environmental pollution increases the risk of pollen allergies.

Studies have shown that the ozone concentration in the air does indeed have an influence on the allergenic activity of pollen. Today we have methods for measuring the concentration of individual allergens in pollen (for experts: Sandwich ELISA using monoclonal antibodies). Grass pollen exposed to a high level of ozone had a higher level of an important allergen (see p. 30 for a discussion of the main allergens) than pollen that was not exposed to ozone. This research is still in its infancy, but it is clear here too that the proper thing to do – throughout the world – is to fight the increase of ozone in the atmosphere. The increase of ozone in the air at certain times of the year may be one reason why there has also been an increase in the number of persons with allergies. The University of Paderborn in Germany has chosen as its main research topic the connection between ozone concentration and the allergenicity of pollen. We now (patiently) await their results, which I certainly hope to present in, say, the 10th edition of this book.

A Japanese study demonstrated that people living in an area of high diesel exhaust pollution but relatively low airborne pollen are more often allergic to the pollen than those living in areas of dense pollen but no diesel pollution. Extensive studies are being carried out as well, but as far as I know, there are as yet no conclusive results, and entirely new aspects are under discussion (see pp. 56–59).

Pollen allergies and your date of birth

Swedish studies have shown that babies born during the birch pollen season are more often allergic to birch than babies born at other times of the year. So, mothers and fathers to be: Don't forget to keep that pollen calendar in mind when "getting down to it"!

House dust mites and other perennial allergens

After pollen allergies, perennial allergies are the main players in the allergy drama. Perennial allergens, i. e., those present all year round, consist mainly of house dust and storage mites, animal hair, molds, and food. The primary perennial allergens are house dust mites such as *Dermatophagoides pteronyssinus* and *Dermatophagoides farinae*, tiny arachnids prevalent in house dust.

Studies have shown that in Hamburg (my home town) the allergic reaction to house dust mites lies around 14%, in Erfurt (a city in eastern Germany) it is 10%. Data from Hamburg, Beelitz, Essen, Bochum and Marburg show that of the 3200 persons investigated, 26% were allergic to house dust mites and 10% to storage mites (see also p. 21). Mites are arachnids that often occur in house dust. Figure 5 shows a "father-mother-child" trio of house dust mites devouring

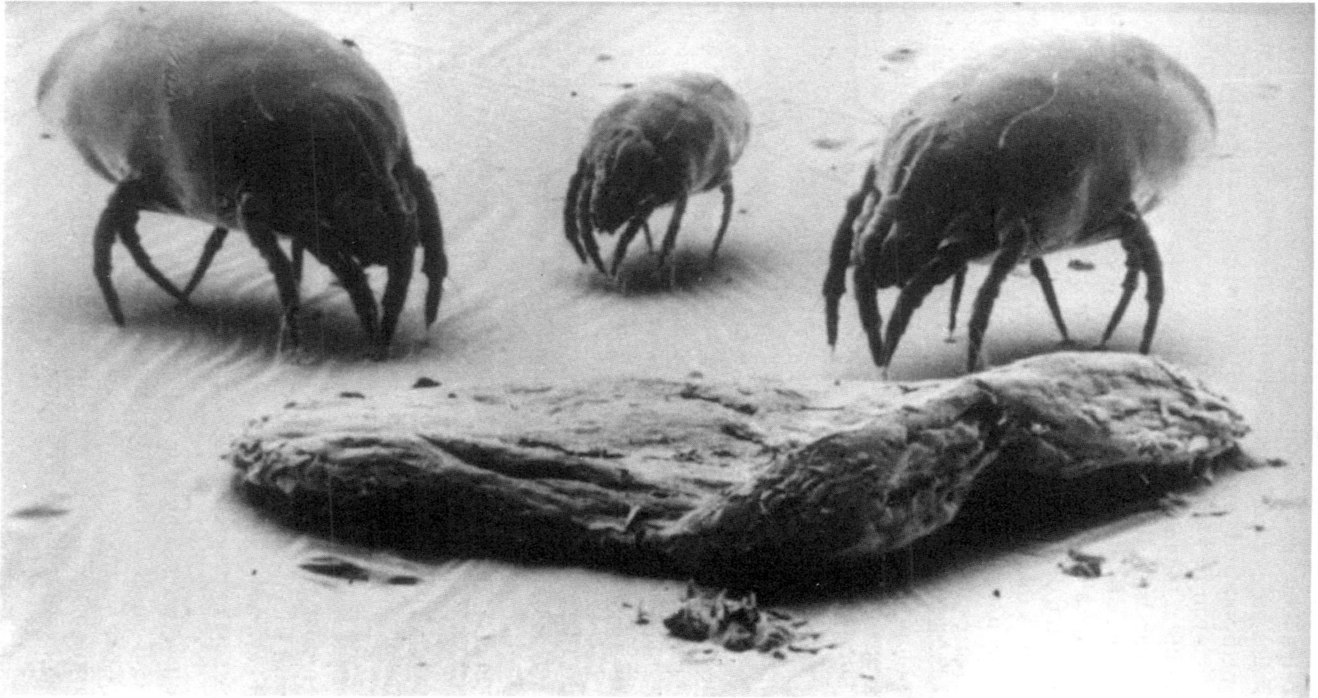

Figure 5. A "mite family" devouring a skin scale as seen under an electron microscope. Dig in, kids, plenty more where that came from!

skin scales, their favorite food, as seen under an electron microscope. Skin scales are present extensively throughout the home, primarily in the bedroom and particularly in beds, where over 60% of all house dust mites can be found. As their presence, unfortunately, does not depend upon the materials from which mattresses and bedding are made, there is no logical reason to change to synthetic fibers. Synthetic materials, including foam mattresses, offer no protection because skin scales abound there just the same, supplying our little friends with a delicious meal. Mite contamination is usually lower in feather beds than in those made from synthetic materials. To think how many mites I once threw at my brother and sister in our pillow fights makes me dizzy. Bedrooms offer house dust mites sufficient food (skin scales), ideal temperatures (20°C or 68°F) and high humidity (approx. 80%). One million house dust mites can "gorge themselves" on one gram of skin scales for an entire week. Human beings lose about 1.5 grams of skin scale per day, thus ensuring a plentiful food supply.

House dust mites have 8 legs, no eyes, and live for approx. 3–4 months, during which time a female lays about 300 eggs. These mite are the most aggressive allergen in house dust. Patients with a particular predisposition can develop serious allergies, or even bronchial asthma. American studies have shown that 45% of young people with this type of asthma are allergic to house dust mites.

Around 100 house dust mites are found per gram of dust in mattresses, whereas only about 10 are found in this amount of dust on the floor. In occupied apartments, the number of house dust mites can vary between 10 and more than 1000 critters per gram of dust. The prevalence of house dust mites in dust can be investigated with the help of a readily available, easy-to-use test strip which determines the amount of guanine, excreted by house dust mites, in house dust.

No matter how lonely and depressed you might feel, you are never alone in bed: your tiny mite friends are always with you. Luckily for you, your friends are so tiny (0.3 mm across) they are invisible to the naked eye – what a horrible, nightmarish thought if this weren't so! But rest assured, ten mites could fit onto this point: •

Mites have been sighted on old tennis balls and stuffed animals as well. Is it possible that the grunting sounds Monica Seles used to make when serving were merely an allergic reaction to the mites in her tennis balls? Who knows. (Does she still grunt like she used to? Haven't heard from her in a while.)

Since mites can be found in house dust all year round, people with this type of allergy suffer much more than people who are allergic to pollen.

In addition to house dust mites, there are also storage mites *(Acarus siro, Tyrophagus putrescentiae, Lepidoglyphus destructor)*, mainly found in the countryside, and as the name suggests, in places where food is stored. But the feed of small animals such as hamsters and gerbils may also be breeding spots for mites. Allergic reactions to hay dust and threshing dust can also be caused by such storage mites, something to keep in mind if you notice horses reacting allergically to straw. Animals, too, are allergic to various substances – just like us. Storage mites thrive on mold, which is one reason why they are so prevalent in houses and apartments prone to having mold. Thus, one should also test for storage mites when testing for mold (see *in vivo/in vitro,* pp. 85–92).

Then there are predatory mites *(Chyletus eruditus)*, who prey on the house dust mites. Why, you might ask, don't we simply set these predatory mites loose on the house dust mites so that the prime allergens in house dust are destroyed? A nice thought, but as predatory mites cause allergies as well, we would simply be jumping from the frying pan into the fire.

House dust mites and rock 'n' roll

Endearing characters that they are, house dust mites have even inspired famous rock musicians:

- The Rolling Stones: Let's spend the mite together
- Art Garfunkel: Mite eyes
- Manfred Mann: Mite y Quin
- Elvis Presley: One mite with you
  Are you lonesome two mites
- Ten Years After: Feeling all mite alright
- Tina Turner: Mite bush city
- The Beatles: Ticket to mites
- Frank Sinatra: Strangers in the mite
- John Travolta: Saturday mite fever
- The Moody Blues: Mites in white satin (They knew!)
- Free: All mite now
- Steppenwolf (60's hippie-band): Born to be mite
- Bee Gees (barf): Saturday mite fever

Remember Bob Dylan's words: It's all mite, Ma, I'm only bleeding.

Cole Porter wrote a little more obliquely with "I've got you under my skin" and even Andrew Lloyd Webber paid homage to the rollerskating mite with "Starmite express." I'd be happy to accept any further suggestions or contributions until August 25, 2030.

I too was kissed by the allergy muse and have written 15 songs with guitar accompaniment, such as the hit "The Allergic Patient," "The Lonely Scientist" (a song that speaks from my heart, Fig. 6) or *the* hymn to all allergy sufferers: "Airborne Pollen" (Fig. 7). I have always imagined arranging this piece for classical instrumentation. If you should have any ideas on this, send me your arrangement. Maybe we'll make a record or CD, become famous and receive the Golden Pollen from the "Pollen information service"! Let's not forget to include the allergy rock 'n' roll song "Am I Allergic." I play it in E major with a good, grooving rock 'n' roll rhythm, although it could also be rapped. Here are the lyrics:

Am I allergic?

Doctor, doctor, won't you help me,
I can't take it anymore,
I've just got to get out of the house –
First the cat and then the dog,
Now it's the flowers, they're much too bright
Am I allergic?

I crawled along the floor and chased the house dust mite,
But unfortunately they were all much too small
I only bought synthetics and Acarosan.
Don't I have it hard?
Am I allergic?
Refrain

These critters always find a way
to plague me and to spoil my day
Am I allergic?

I let them prick me in the belly
and then in the arm as well,
A rash was nothing new for me,
I knew all the doctors in this town,
And oh, was I allergologically known.
Am I allergic?
Refrain

During pollen season I escaped to Helgoland,

And avoided house dust at all cost,
People all around were having fun
And I was socially completely lost
Am I allergic?
Refrain

Is it the car exhaust or maybe
the cigar smoke, can it come
from merely breathing?
Is it my hair or possibly my belly
or is it all psychosomatic?
Am I allergic?

These critters always find a way
to plague me and to spoil my day
Am I allergic?

Oh, I've accepted it all in the end,
but my next rash is just round the bend.
I'm allergic, oh yeah
I'm allergic, oh yeah

THE LONELY SCIENTIST

Text & Musik: Rüdiger Wahl
Bearbeitung: Werner Lang

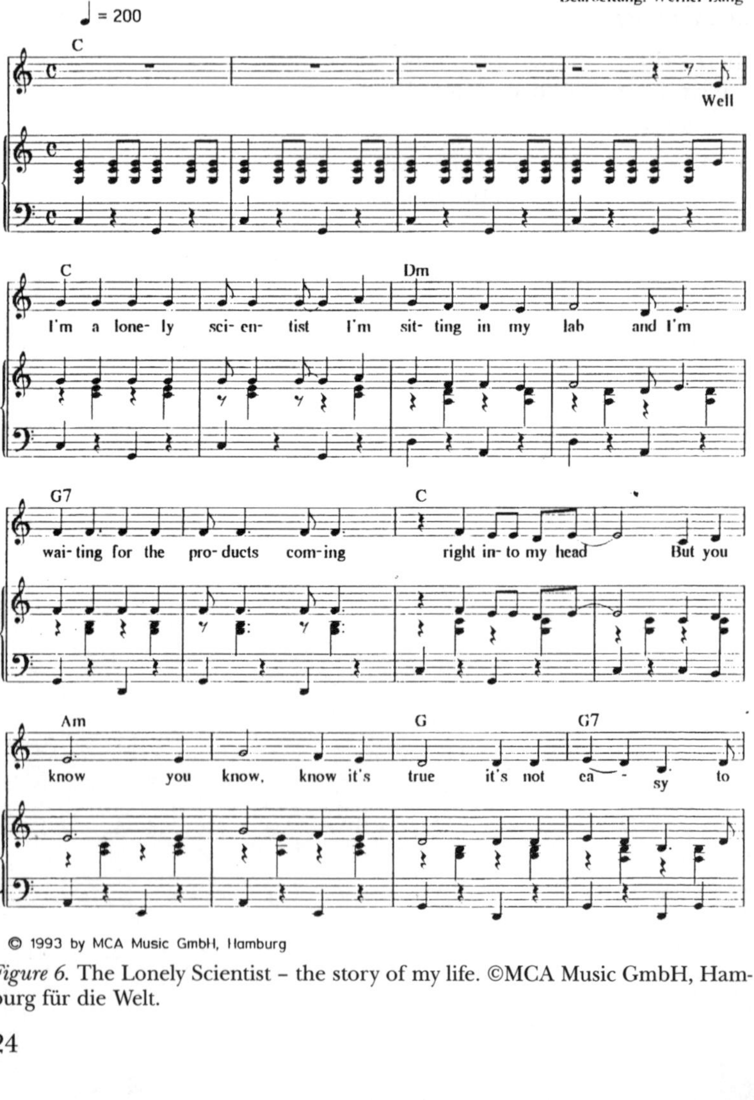

© 1993 by MCA Music GmbH, Hamburg

Figure 6. The Lonely Scientist – the story of my life. ©MCA Music GmbH, Hamburg für die Welt.

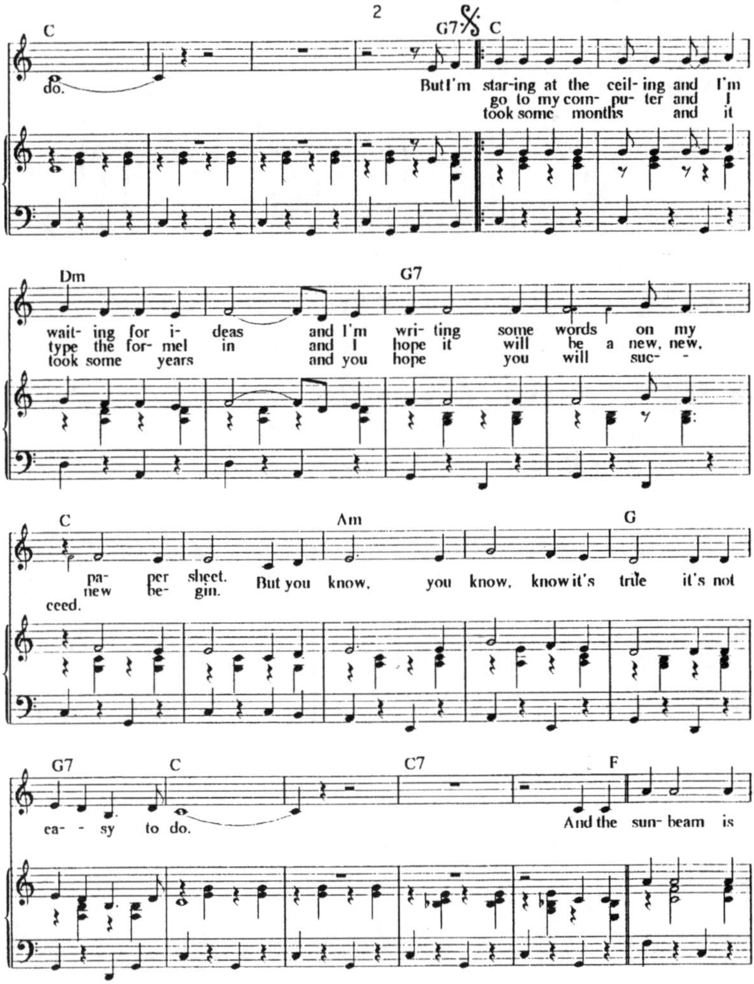

Figure 6. The Lonely Scientist (continued)

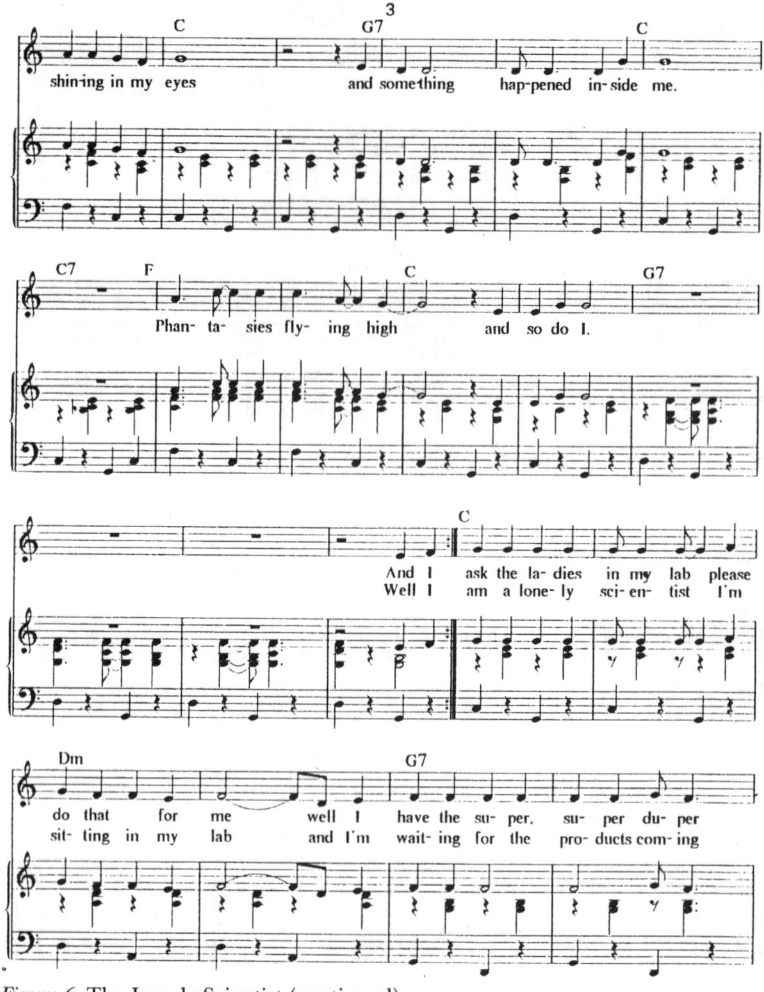

Figure 6. The Lonely Scientist (continued)

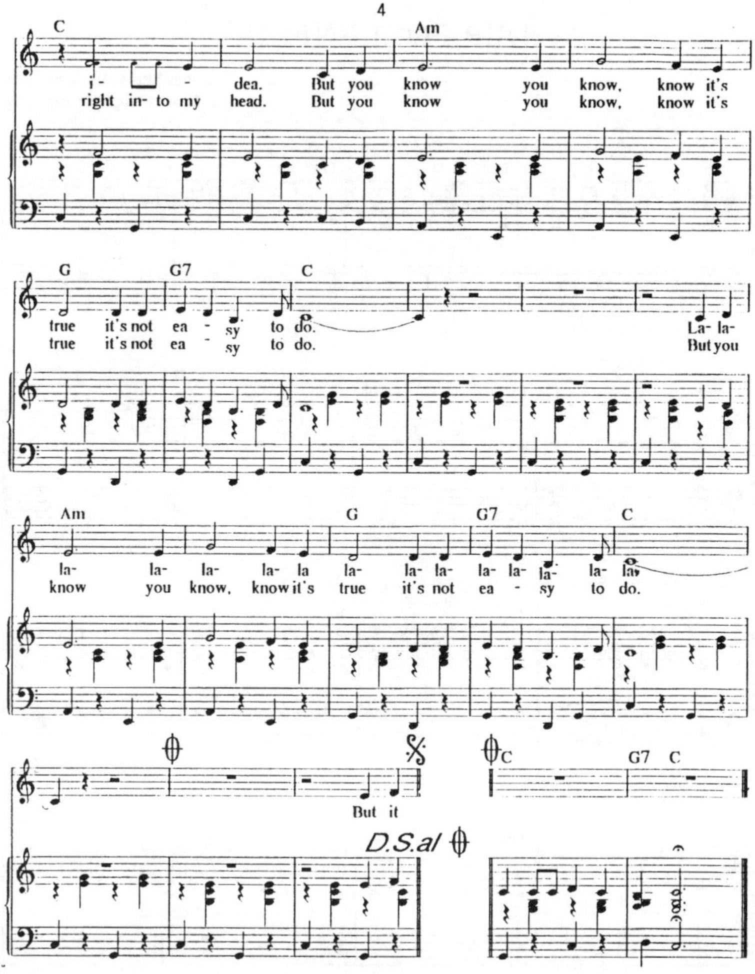

Figure 6. The Lonely Scientist (continued)

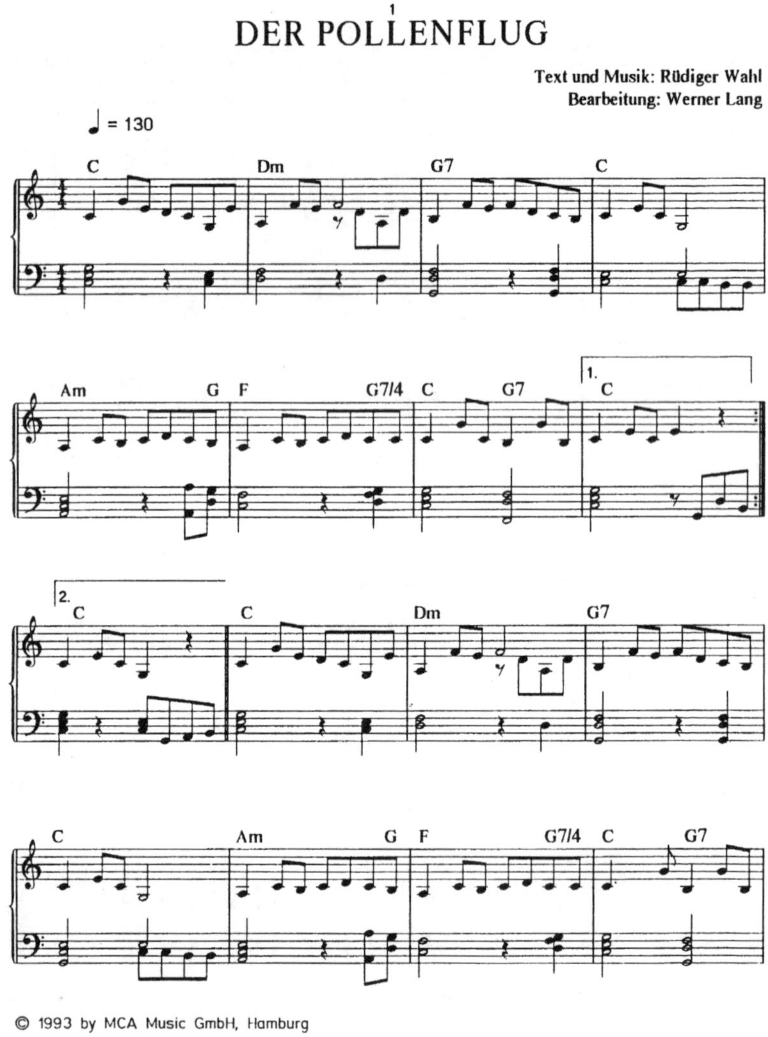

Figure 7. "Airborne Pollen" – actually written for guitar. This is the piano version, which isn't bad either. ©MCA Music GmbH, Hamburg für die Welt.

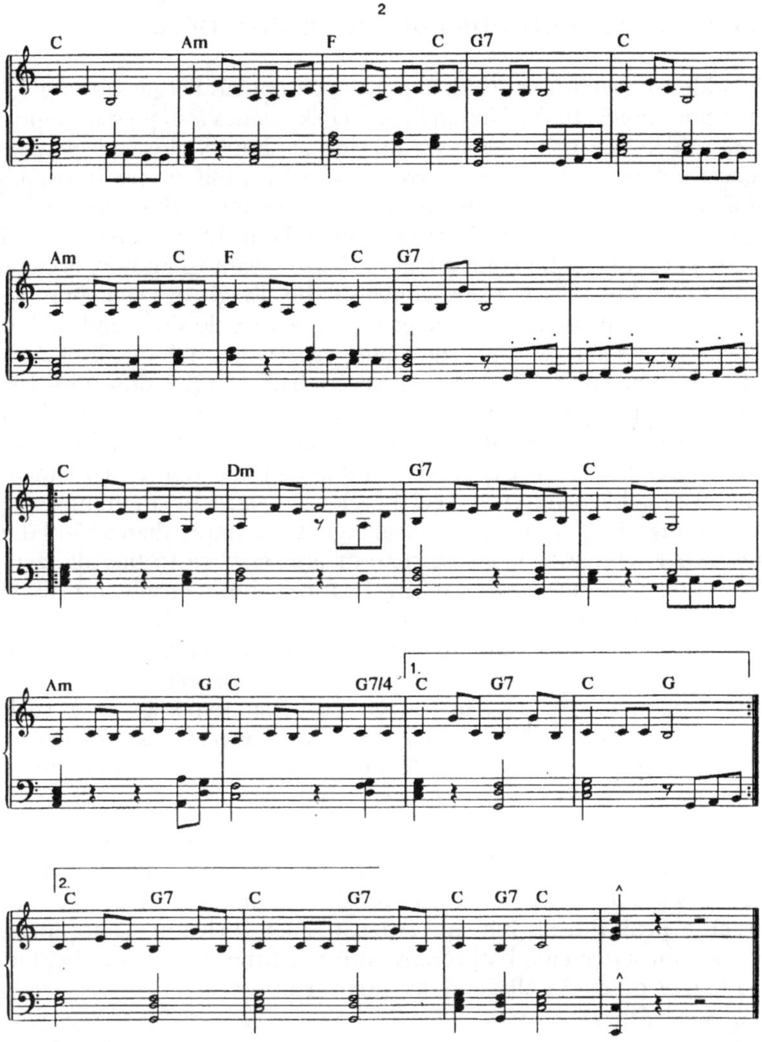

Figure 7. Airborne pollen (continued)

What other perennial allergens are there?

In addition to mites, the most important perennial allergens are animal hair and molds. In the United States, cockroaches also play an important role in house dust allergy. And German households – please take a seat before reading this – have a total of 7.8 million pet birds, 3.5 million other small animals such as hamsters and gerbils, 3.1 million aquariums with literally millions of fish in them, 4.8 million dogs, and 5.5 million cats (who counted all of these, I want to know?). So, our houses are just full of diverse animals to be allergic to – not counting of course all the plastic baby alligators, Lacoste polo shirts and rubber duckies. Cats and dogs are the main perpetrators indoors. In 9–41% of all asthma sufferers, skin tests for cat hair allergies show positive. The main allergen in cats is in fact their saliva, and when they clean themselves, they distribute it nicely all over their fur. Cat hair, in turn, distributes this "saliva allergen" throughout the house. This main allergen has been designated Fel d 1 (*Felis domesticus* or common house cat). Many allergens contain main allergens, i. e., more than 50% of the respective allergic persons react to or are sensitive to this allergen. When a cat grooms itself by licking its fur, it automatically spreads its saliva and thus the saliva allergen as well. It is relatively unknown for specific breeds of cats to cause allergic reactions but this is often the case with dogs. In part, research has shown that people allergic to cats react more strongly to normal "street cats" than to pedigree cats such as Persian or Siamese. That topic should be worth at least a couple of doctoral dissertations from up and coming scientists. Further animal allergies will be discussed on pages 35 and 48.

Mold species such as *Alternaria tenuis, Cladosporium herbarum, Penicillium notatum* etc. – not to be confused with edible molds such as those found on mushrooms – are considered perennial allergens, but reach a peak during July and August. They thrive in damp apartments, musty cellars, bathrooms with too little ventilation, behind wallpaper on cold walls, and on rotten fruit.

*A patient was having allergic reactions upon repotting his flowers. Various immunobiochemical tests revealed that it was not the potting soil, but the mold contained therein (*Clacosporium herbarum *in this case) that was causing the problem.*

As molds have even been discovered in the soil of potted plants, people allergic to molds should always wear gloves when repotting, or better still let someone else do the job as the mold allergens can also be inhaled. Feeling unwell in an air-conditioned room could also indicate an allergy to mold. The particle size of the mold spores lies between 2 and 4 micrometers.

The incidence of allergic reactions to mold is viewed differently depending on which allergy outpatient facility you consult, with the rates given said to lie between 1% and 30%. The most important molds causing allergic reactions are *Alternaria tenius, Cladosporium herbarum, Aspergillus fumigatus* and *Penicillium notatum*.

Dust is a perennial allergen too, but here we are not dealing with a single "pure" substance such as pollen or mite but an extremely heterogeneous mixture of mites, cockroaches, animal hair, pollen, molds, insects, food particles, etc. Nonetheless, house dust mites are still the most important allergens in house dust.

The dust from households without animals of any sort still contain animal allergens such as those from dogs and cats. These allergens are transported into the living spaces on our clothes and shoes. If the result for mites from a test for house dust allergy is negative, then one should test for animal epithelia, even if there are no animals present in the household. One should also consider the plants present, such as *Ficus benjamina*, when testing for house dust allergy.

What can you do if you're allergic to house dust mites?

As we know, house dust mites are impossible to see with the naked eye. Using a magnifying glass won't do either, unfortunately, and crawling around the house with a microscope would be very tiring and impractical (Fig. 8). So how can we fight this invisible enemy? We are unable to prevent the human skin from shedding and cannot thus cut off the parasite's principle food supply, so we must seek other methods of mite genocide. I have included a list of such measures, added to which you could store your bedding in a big chest freezer (sweet dreams) or cram it into the oven (careful not to brown to quickly), or use any readily available anti-mite spray on your mattress, upholstery, and carpets in order to kill the mites, lump them together and vacuum them up. You can also trap the parasites in mite-proof mattress or duvet covers and pillowcases. Research has shown that this method drastically reduces allergic attacks against mites. Buy a new mattress beforehand to keep the mite population as low as possible from the outset and let a non-allergic person dispose of your bedding.

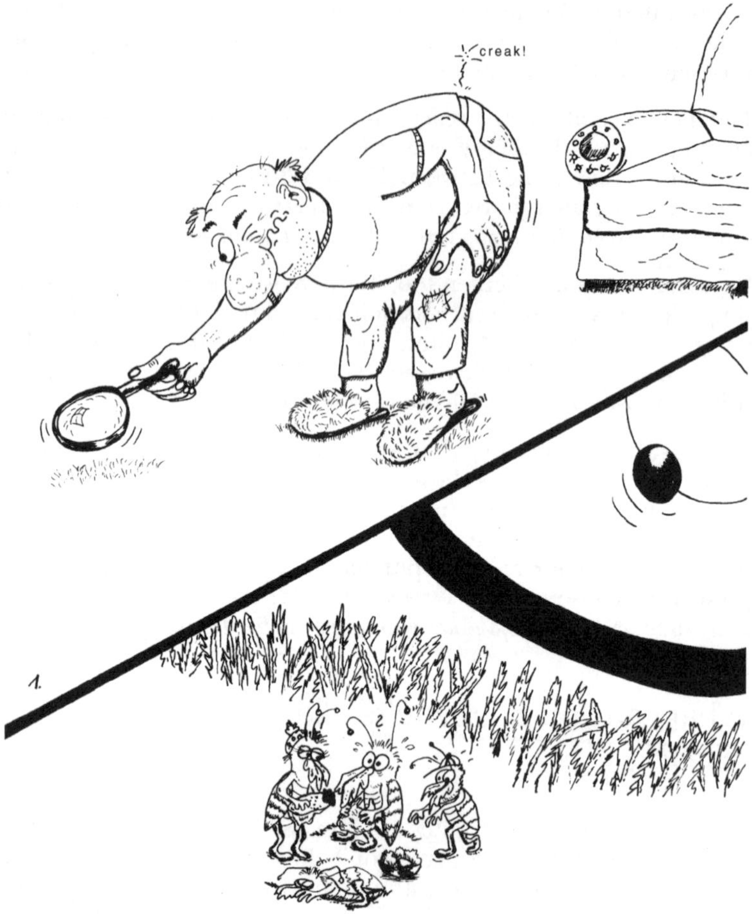

Figure 8. Come out, come out, wherever you are!

Proper ventilation is also helpful. The rule is that an hour with the window completely open is better than 24 hours of a slightly opened window.

The chaotic person who leaves the bed unmade is, in one respect, doing a better job fighting mites than the pedantic bedmaker who always leaves things orderly and, to top it off, pulls the bedspread neatly over the entire bed, puts the pillows on top and marks a crease in the middle. But the chaotic person tends to make the mistake of putting the mattress directly on the floor, which is an invitation to mites to move in, whereas the pedantic person always has to have a bedcase. So it's a draw. Decide for yourself where you fit in here. I myself am more of a chaotic person, especially if my wife weren't watching out for me.

Sanitizing the bed is an important matter for people who are allergic to mites; as mentioned, mites can easily reproduce under the ideal conditions present in a mattress. Usually everything is infiltrated – the mattress, the sheets, and the blankets. The use of extra sheets or duvet covers keeps the mites trapped within the mattress and duvet – and no mites can invade them from the outside and lay their eggs. Also, these special sheets are often accepted by health-insurance companies as protection against house dust mites, and because they are made of a rugged special fabric, they last a long time.

In order to reduce the number of mites in your surroundings, you have to pay special attention to bed hygiene. This means, first, washing bed linen at high temperatures of 60 to 95°C (140 to 195°F) since mite eggs are killed off only at 95°C (195°F). Washing bed linen weekly reduces the amount of foodstuffs available to the the mites (such as skin scales). Special attention should be paid to places where skin is exposed, such as pillows and at the foot end of the bed – which is also where the most skin scales are lost, providing mites with an ideal environment. Many of the extra sheets and covers mentioned above have a very smooth surface, but that doesn't mean you'll slide off the bed: These special sheets should obviously be covered with your normal sheets and blankets or pillow cases.

Today, powerful apparatus are also available for filtering out allergenic matter from the air, such as pollen and mites, which makes the air much more pleasant for the allergic person to breath. The costs for these mattress covers and filter apparatus are often paid for by health insurance. It's at least worth an inquiry with your carrier.

Another solution would be to have yourself hyposensitized (see p. 93) or to move to the Antarctic where you'll most definitely be safe, right? (Fig. 9).

Don't worry, you don't have to go quite that far. House dust mites have been proven non-existent in textile dust at altitudes of over 5,000 feet (around 1,500 meters). In such areas, the long, hard winters dry out your home to such an extent that no mite could possibly survive. Just think, by romping in the snow and going skiing you avoid house dust mites – just as long as you don't venture below 5,000 feet where they'll be lining up to attack! A side note on skiing: I attempted to learn to ski at a rather advanced age, but instead of spending time on the slopes, I ended up nursing my bandaged limbs or running over other skiers, since I simply couldn't find the brakes. Back at my

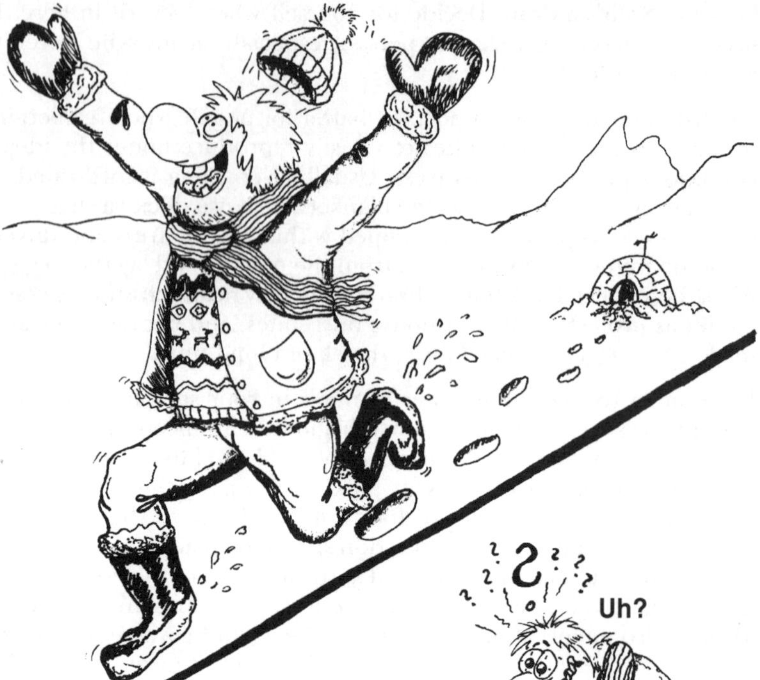

Figure 9. Thank goodness, no more mites. Brrr, it's cold here – What's thaaaat? Uh?

hotel I seriously began to wonder whether going skiing was really a vacation or a masochistic event. Since I myself am not allergic to mites, I really and truly do not need to go to the Alps, but will stay at the oceanside where I belong.

As you can see, there are many ways of making a mite's life hard and/or escaping them. But house dust mite allergies certainly limit your enjoyment of life and if you're allergic, you endure great suffering all year round.

What can you do if you're allergic to cat and dog hair?

The simplest thing would be to give the animal away, but for some this could go beyond the pain threshold. If your cat has been a long-standing member of the family (mine died when it was 20, which is around 120 in cat years) with whom you've shared many joys and sorrows and you're dead set on keeping – there's always the option illustrated in Figure 10. Bathe or shower your cat once a week, and you will greatly reduce the number of offending allergens like Fel d 1. Desensitizing your own person could seriously improve your chances of not having to part with the pet at all, but failing that, you'll have to find your own way of getting the animal under the shower without the help of catnip shampoo (sadly not yet on the market). The risk involved here is that your beloved puss may suddenly take a lightning decision to forthwith abandon the domestic security you provide and take its chances in the Great Outdoors. The fact remains, and has been scientifically proven, that bathing your cat once a week vastly reduces the allergens. My cat refuses to let itself even be brushed, but it's probably all a matter of what it's used to. Good luck, and for pity's sake don't leave it to a "lick and a promise."

If you're allergic to cats and are planning to move into a new apartment, make sure the previous tenant didn't have any. Research has shown that although a cat may not have inhabited an apartment for many years, cat allergens can still be clearly detected. In any case you will have to repaint and repaper the apartment, lay new carpets, etc., and then – if you feel the need – you can always buy a porcelain cat – guaranteed to be allergy-free, easy to care for, but a dust trap. Watch out if you're allergic to dust!

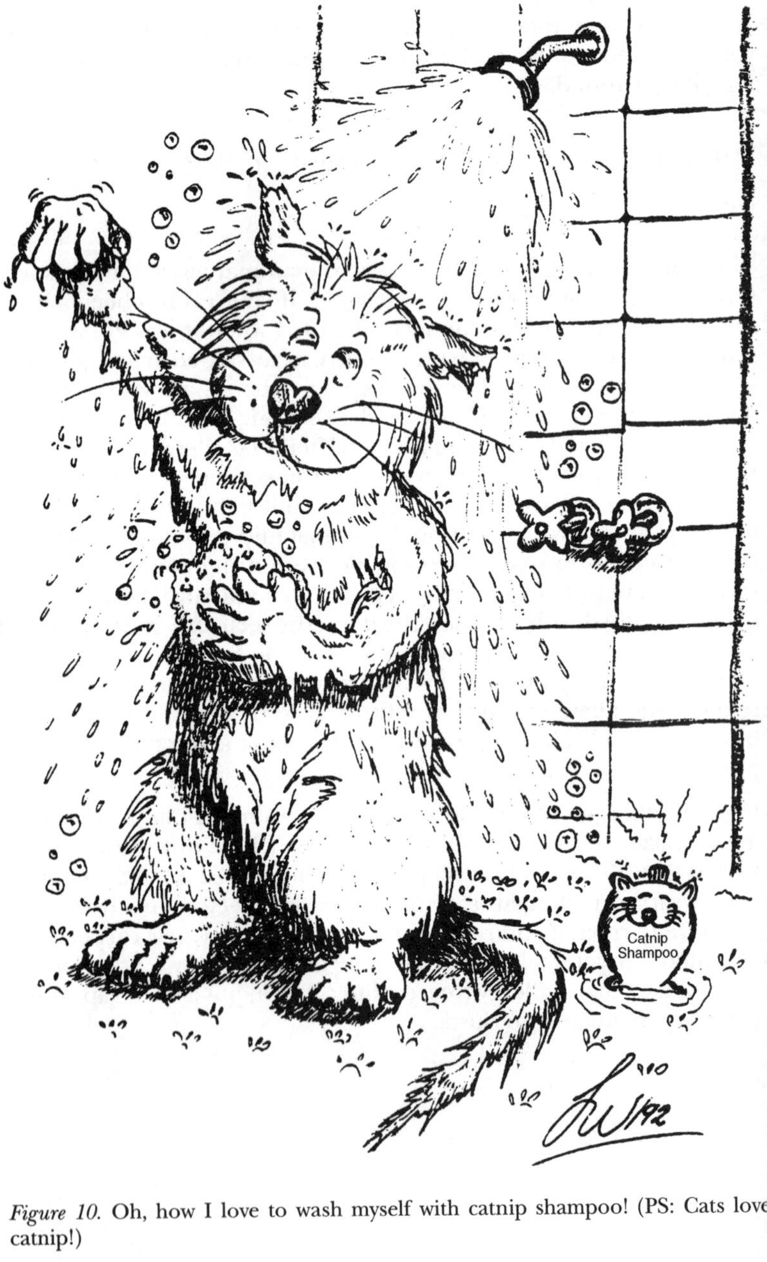

Figure 10. Oh, how I love to wash myself with catnip shampoo! (PS: Cats love catnip!)

Allergies in the classroom

Allergic to school? That's nothing new, but not what I want to discuss. Nearly all of us have gone through such phases or are experiencing them now but don't necessarily have to. On a more serious note, people prone to allergies can suffer badly at school. A Swedish study revealed that cat and dog hair can be so prevalent in classrooms as to trigger asthma in certain people. Teachers and students carry the allergens to school in their clothing. The allergens then find their most stable residence on the chairs, largely because they are far less frequently cleaned than desks and floors.

For no apparent reason at first, a boy began to suffer serious allergies in his classroom. After a while, concentration focused on a stuffed animal which had been brought up from the cellar and placed in the classroom for decoration. Because of its long term of residence in a damp cellar, the animal had grown a mold, and it so happened that the child was allergic to this substance. The stuffed animal was removed and the student's allergic reaction vanished.

If children develop allergic reactions at school, the first step should be to check whether or not allergens such as animal hair are being brought into the school. As we have seen, however, other sources, like stuffed animals often used in biology classes, can also cause allergies. Food particles shouldn't be forgotten, either. According to one Norwegian study, substantial amounts of smoked salmon were found in classroom dust, triggering allergic reactions in predisposed children. The smoked salmon particles came from the children's packed lunches which in Norway often feature smoked salmon sandwiches.

Allergies and insects

Not only bees and wasps but a variety of insects can cause allergies in predisposed patients. In the United States, for instance, most people suffering from perennial allergies react strongly to cockroaches (*Blatella germanica* and *Periplaneta americana*). For reasons more to do with the beauty of their name than their penchant for causing allergies, the Spanish song "La Cucaracha" sings their praises. There is even a (rather unsavoury) book about cockroaches attacking human beings, and although it did not deal with the subject of **this** book, allergies too can attack and seriously interfere with our enjoyment of life!

The major insect allergens in the United States are those of the red ant. No cases of an allergic reaction to this ant poison are known to me from Germany – but perhaps you know some.

An allergy of particular significance for people living in houses with renovated attics is the pigeon tick allergy. These insects occur mainly in old buildings with attics. When the attics are cleaned out, the pigeons scatter but the ticks remain. Having lost their host, the insects migrate downward through the building in search of a new host. Allergic reactions to pigeon ticks can even result in anaphylactic shock.

A further insect allergy I mustn't forget is the house fly allergy.

Upon coming into contact with a house fly, a farmer's wife noticed a reddening of her eye. As the wings of the fly brushed her eye, the patient immediately reacted with conjunctivitis. In vitro tests (see p. 88) indicated that the patient's serum contained the specific IgE against flies. The combination of in vivo and in vitro tests confirmed that she was seriously allergic to flies. In such cases a fly swatter could be appropriate, but flies must be avoided as much as possible. Since the patient lived and worked on a farm, this was very difficult to do, but she managed to hang flyproof cloth across her windows and reduced the amount of time she spent in the barn.

Although controversial discussion is still raging as to whether silver fish in house dust can cause allergic reactions, their allergenic potency appears to be rather minimal. You can breed them on paper tissues soaked in sugar water and left at high humidity. But why would anyone want to do such a thing?

A Trogoderma allergy was discovered in Berlin, Germany; the patient reported allergic responses whenever he approached his apartment on the fifth floor of the building. They disappeared when he visited a woman downstairs on the first floor. One might suggest the easiest solution would be for him to simply move in – for purely therapeutic reasons – with the female neighbor even though it is both likely and reasonable that such a "simple" solution would have resulted in marital strife. Happily, investigations proved that the woman downstairs played no role at all, the cause was the Trogoderma beetle found in his apartment but not in hers. In the light of this discovery, telling your wife that you have to run downstairs to see the woman on the other floor to obtain relief from your allergies, will not really stand as a convincing argument.

Allergic reactions to insects is an area, as yet, still wide open for study. To date, relatively few allergy-causing insects have been documented, and the allergenic source is for the most part unknown. Is it their bodies, their poison, their saliva? Or is it the dirt they pick up when eating?

In the case of bees and wasps, the main allergenic source has been found to be their poison.

What are allergens?

Now that we have heard so much about allergens, its time to clear up what they actually are. Nearly any material or substance can affect a patient with a particular predisposition. Allergens are primarily made up of proteins. Pollen, house dust mites, animal epithelia, food, med-

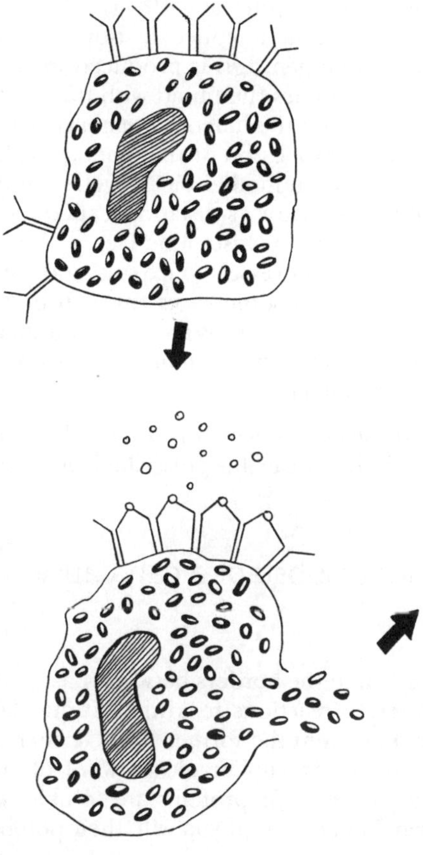

Figure 11. Allergen (o), IgE (Y), mast cell (above) and release of histamine from the mast cell (below).

ication, etc., can all act as allergens. Such substances are introduced from outside the body through inhalation, skin contact, oral ingestion, or injection, as with an insect bite.

What happens when an allergen enters your body?

To explain what happens when an allergen enters your body, it is unfortunately necessary to get a little technical. When allergens enter an organism, the organism responds by producing antibodies. Immunoglobulin E (IgE) plays the largest role in the allergic reactions of the early types. It becomes obvious that the study of allergies is a very recent science when you consider that IgE was only discovered by Johansson and Ishizaka (who deserve the Nobel Prize in my mind) as late as 1967. One reason for its being so hard to detect is that compared to other antibodies, it is present in very low concentration, i.e., only 17–450 ng/ml (billionths of a gram, 50×10^{-9} g), whereas Immunoglobulin G (IgG) is present at a concentration of 8–16 mg/ml. Upon contact with the allergen, IgE is produced in the plasma cells in our blood. These antibodies then bind with the mast cells (Fig. 11). Mast cells are found under the mucous membranes in the body such as the nose, lungs and eyes. Upon further contact with the allergen – pollen, for instance – the antibodies bind together and the cells release a multitude of inflammatory substances called mediators. One example of these mediators is histamine (see p. 106). The release of histamine can cause blood vessels to expand and can result in acute allergic inflammation. In some cases this can even lead to tissue damage or asthma. As the mast cells are located under the mucous membranes, allergic reactions will result in a runny nose (rhinitis) or red, streaming eyes (conjunctivitis).

In order to inhibit the release of histamine which is responsible for various symptoms, antihistamine drugs can be prescribed by your doctor.

How do you tell whether a substance can cause allergies?

This was illustrated quite simply when the borders between East and West Germany opened up. Allergic reactions to kiwi fruit and latex (see p. 66) were basically unknown in the former East Germany. Kiwis were not available in stores and rubber gloves were often washed and reused due to their scarcity. As proteins are soluble in water, rinsing the "latex allergens" decreased, if you will, their potency. Now, by contrast, due to the risk of infection for patients, doctors and nurses, rubber gloves in both parts of Germany are only worn once and then destroyed. Doctors and other hospital staff are the prime target group as they are likely to sensitize themselves through regular contact with the allergens. In the United States 14% of hospital staff are allergic to latex and in Germany 8.9%. Any company succeeding in manufacturing gloves of the same texture and "sensitivity" from a substance other than latex would not only help many allergy sufferers but become rich overnight! So scientists, roll up your sleeves and get to work! The latex jackpot's waiting!

But back to the kiwi: What do kiwis have to do with the fall of the Berlin wall? When the borders opened, the former East Germany was forced to take the bad with the good. One of the advantages was that stores now stocked various types of fruit like papaya, passion fruit and kiwi. Because they are high in vitamin C, kiwis became popular overnight and are now as common in the East as they were in the West. It wasn't long, however, before the first kiwi allergies appeared. This fruit has a high potential for allergens, and although I am non-atopic (see p. 54), I notice, after eating a kiwi, a distinctly itchy feeling in my throat. Even the inhabitants of the former West Germany are obviously not safe! Then again, not many years ago we too considered kiwis an exotic fruit which, once it had appeared on the market, caused severe allergies in predisposed patients.

On a flight to Washington several years ago to attend a conference at the "American Academy of Clinical Immunology and Allergy," one of the passengers had an extreme allergic reaction after eating yogurt. The plane was forced to make an emergency landing and the woman was given medical attention. This same woman, interestingly enough, turned out to be a speaker at the congress, where she later told us that her allergic reaction had been caused by the kiwi in the yogurt. She hadn't known, previously, that she was allergic to kiwis which goes to show just how aggressive the allergens in that particular fruit can be.

Now back to our actual subject: Is it possible that such "isolated phenomena" can explain allergic reactions to house dust mites? According to studies from Papua New Guinea, the answer is: yes. Although the inhabitants of Papua New Guinea used to sleep on the ground, this did not stop civilization from introducing one of its "benefits": the mattress, offering people a softer bed, but simultaneously providing ideal conditions for house dust mites. Indeed, before very long the first house dust mite allergies began to appear.

These examples prove the allergenic potency of various substances which primarily affect atopic individuals (see p. 54).

They also show, as history has so often proved, that civilization introduces not only advantages but disadvantages, as the inhabitants of Papua New Guinea experienced when "civilized" with the mattress which in turn becomes colonized by the mites.

What medical conditions are caused by allergies?

The most widespread are asthma and hay fever, followed by general forms of urticaria, which manifest themselves in swelling and reddening of the skin. We should also mention contact dermatitis, the irritation that can occur when the body comes in contact with an allergen.

> *A patient who loved wearing skintight jeans [as I did in my youth, although I have to go for the "loose" or "comfortable" fit nowadays like Dockers] developed a rash right where the top button pressed against her bellybutton. This turned out to be a classic case of nickel allergy combined with contact dermatitis.*

Thanks to fashion, males are no less prone to nickel allergies than females. Just wearing an earring containing nickel can lead to the discovery of an allergy that necessitate a change of job. You want an example? An auto mechanic, of course, as his work would entail frequent handling of materials with significant nickel content.

What do women unable to afford gold or platinum jewellery do? Simply tell their loved ones they have developed a nickel allergy and can only survive free of allergies by wearing platinum or gold (what else – after all, diamonds are a girl's best friends – oh Marilyn!).

Asthma is an allergy which can seriously shrink your enjoyment of life, and it has been determined that rhinitis – if untreated – can lead to asthma, first affecting the upper air passages and then the lungs. To prevent such a development, hyposensitization (see p. 93) should be considered in advance.

Neurodermatitis

Many toddlers and school children suffer from this terrible disease also called atopic dermatitis or atopic eczema. In 1993, neurodermatitis was found to affect 12% of school children in the district of Hannover, a city in northern Germany. In the US two million children have eczema (atopic dermatitis). About 5% of allergic people in the UK suffer from atopic dermatitis. Featuring itchiness and scabbing, the disease often disappears as the children grow older. It is said to have various possible causes, one of which is food, such as cow's milk, eggs, sugar, nuts, herbs, spices and (to an increasing degree) soy products. Other causes include house dust mites, as some studies show, and animal hair. Many children take their pets with them to bed, so it is vital to check for animal hair in the bedroom. As with food, the best way to deal with house dust mites and animal hair is to avoid them altogether (see p. 92). Mattresses and bedding can be covered with special, mite-proof material which offers some protection. Pets cannot be treated like a Christo art event and wrapped up, so they have to go – a painful solution, but in the end no more painful than the neurodermatitis itself.

In many cases, the disease can be rooted in psychological problems. A child might show physical symptoms in response to its parents' separation, or the parents' frequent arguments, or if the child has problems in kindergarten. In this case parents should seek support and assistance from someone trained in educational psychology.

Planning the sensitized child's diet according to the food it is allowed to eat is also necessary, and to prove solidarity and set a good example, parents should themselves try, if possible, to give up things like chocolate which their child is not allowed.

Cortisone is often prescribed to relieve neurodermatitis, something which is unfortunately often viewed in a very negative light. But just think for a minute how many human lives – not only asthma victims – have been saved by cortisone. The drug should only be administered, of course, according to a physician's orders.

Psychological assistance, appropriate diet, and avoiding allergens as well as the right attitude toward drugs, is the best way to relieve neurodermatitis.

Job-related asthma

Job-related asthma is caused by substances a patient frequently encounters in the course of his or her work. Such allergy-causing substances can be divided into seven groups: Platinum salts, isocyanates, epoxy resins and derivates, colophony, proteolytic enzymes, laboratory animals, and flour dust. It is possible to extend this list to include pharmaceutical products, sawdust, raw coffee, and latex. The following is a brief description of the occupations at risk from the above allergens. Figure 12 demonstrates the decisions atopic people are faced with when choosing a career. Although atopic persons are mainly affected, non-atopic people can be sensitized as well, depending on the aggressiveness of the substance. Such sensitization is referred to as an imposed allergy.

Platinum salts	People involved in manufacturing catalytic converters.
Isocyanate	Chemical workers: Isocyanate is used in producing urethane and polyurethane.
Epoxy resins	People involved in manufacturing paints and plastics.
Colophony	Workers in the electrical industry
Proteolytic enzymes	Workers involved in the manufacture of washing powders. Housewives rarely suffer allergic reactions as these enzymes appear in the detergents in encapsulated form.
Laboratory animals	3 to 10% of people in frequent contact with laboratory animals such as rats, rabbits, or mice develop a job-related allergy. The allergen source is usually the urine.
Flour dust	Bakers are the prime victims, although it has to be said that frequently it is other substances in the flour which cause the allergies. These can include the enzyme alpha-amylase or contamination through storage mites, rice bugs *(Tribolium confusum)*, or mold.
Sawdust	Carpenters are especially at risk here although native varieties of wood are not as allergenic as tropical varieties such as teak, mahogany, etc.
Raw coffee	Workers involved in the coffee processing industry and the dockers lugging the bags are mostly affected.
Latex	Allergic reactions to latex are not only triggered by frequent contact with rubber gloves, condoms and balloons (causing swollen lips) but also by inhaling the latex

allergens which stick to the powder on the inside of the gloves. Doctors and other hospital staff are the main sufferers of this allergy. In the United States some hospitals already have latex-free rooms where it is forbidden to work with materials containing latex.

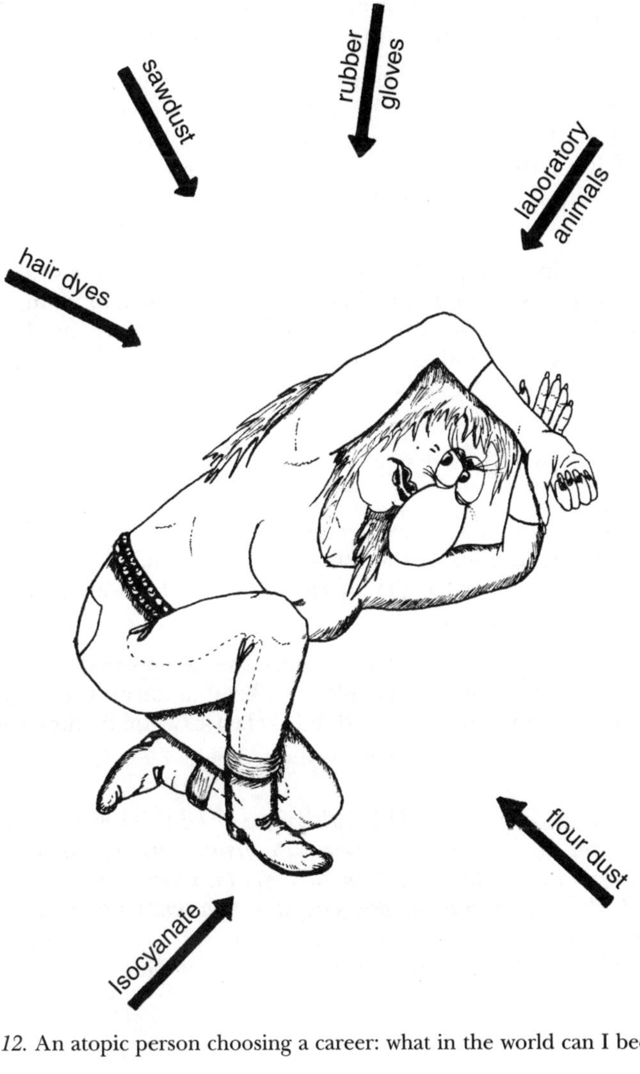

Figure 12. An atopic person choosing a career: what in the world can I become?

Baker's asthma

Flours play a large role in the allergic reactions experienced by bakers. Here, we are dealing with an inhalation allergen. In only some 0.3% of all cases do bakers allergic to flour also react after eating the breads made with those flours – a very small group indeed. The modern trend toward using wholemeal flour to bake with means that other ingredients of high nutritional value such as nuts are included in breads – and likewise provide a source of potential allergens. Some breads today include, for example, amarant, a grain from South Africa.

Studies have shown that bakers who often come in contact with such flours react allergically to them. Runny noses or even asthma can result. One baker's apprentice had difficulty breathing when anywhere within 10 yards of ground amarant flour, which goes to show that amarant is a very powerful allergen indeed. Only the use of face masks and protective clothing can hinder its effects.

Atopic persons (see p. 54) who want to become a baker should first have themselves tested by an allergologist in advance of taking up the job for allergic reactions to flours as inhalation allergens. This may save unnecessary trouble, up to the point of having to get another job.

Allergies and hobbies

Hobbies are intended to give people a relaxing break from their often stressful job situations or sometimes difficult familial ones. But here too, atopic people in particular can sensitize themselves to certain substances and materials.

DIY woodworkers can sensitize themselves to sawdust, particularly that from tropical woods. People who keep aquariums can also develop allergies to water fleas and red fly larvae when feeding the fish.

A fisherman always used bluebottle larvae as bait. Once, after fastening the larva to the hook, he rubbed his eyes and immediately developed conjunctivitis, causing his eyes to redden, stream, and swell. Upon consulting an allergologist, both a skin test and an in vitro test revealed that the fisherman was allergic to bluebottle larvae. He should have used the boring spinner after all!

If shortness of breath, runny nose, streaming eyes, or reddening of the skin occur frequently when practicing your hobbies, the best idea is to contact an allergologist and possibly have a skin test done using the relevant substances to determine the allergens. With certain substances – particularly chemicals – where it is extremely difficult to run an *in vitro* test, an *in vivo* test has to be substituted, which in itself is not always easy. As some substances are toxic, it can be difficult to determine whether the irritation was an allergic reaction or a toxic one. The most effective solution is to take the suspect chemicals to the doctor and have him or her carry out the appropriate tests to determine and identify more precisely what is causing your allergic reaction.

Allergies and fashion

Can nothing stop these allergies, not even fashion? Allergies are not fashionable diseases, in spite of claims to the contrary. Now we are aware that the more intelligent and sensitive members of the population tend to suffer from allergies, it may be considered fashionable to be a little bit allergic as long as it is in no way life-threatening and doesn't interfere too much with one's lifestyle. It has been proven conclusively, however, that fashion is responsible for the *latest* in allergic reactions. Leggins are one example, although at the time of writing they are no longer the hit they once were. (The modern woman now wears stretch pants and, of course, good old jeans, dark blue, not stone-washed, preferably with rivets – but beware the impending nickel allergy!). Leggins are problematic because normal sweating caused particularly by the tight-fitting ones, especially black ones, releases some of the dye in the fabric, which in turn can cause an allergic reaction. So it's back to the hot pants of the 1960s and 1970s, arguably a better sight for macho eyes.

Allergic reactions to medication

Medication is yet another component in the colorful range of allergies, though this is often only a pseudo-allergy: in other words, the symptoms are similar to those of a "normal" allergy but no IgE is produced. In the US nearly 200,000 hospitalized patients suffer allergic drug reactions each year and 50,000 enter the hospital because of them, recent estimates indicate. An example of a genuine allergic reaction to medication is an allergic reaction to penicillin. Patients suffering from such an allergy must avoid penicillin at all cost, as contact with the drug through an injection can lead to the most serious allergic reaction of all: anaphylactic shock. **Anaphylactic shock causes the circulatory system to collapse and must be immediately treated with an injection of adrenaline (epinephrine) which can be done with an auto-injector.** This instrument is the size of a ballpoint pen and very portable. In an emergency, the patient simply injects the medication into the leg through his or her clothing in a matter of seconds. Nevertheless, a doctor should always be contacted immediately. **Typical symptoms of the onset of anaphylactic shock include itchy hands, soles of feet or scalp, sudden drop in blood pressure, swelling of the face and airways, and difficulty breathing.**

Allergic reactions to insect poison

The common stinging insects belong to the order Hymenoptera (of which there are over 16,000 species in North America) and can be divided into families, the apids, which include honeybees and bumblebees; and the vespids, which include yellow jackets, hornets and wasps. Of the two, apids are less aggressive than vespids, but will sting when provoked. There are also several stinging ants which can be considered as non-winged Hymenoptera. The fire ant is a major cause of allergic reactions in the southeastern United States, and the harvester ant is responsible for similar problems in the Southwestern United States.

As the poison enters the bloodstream immediately, people who are allergic to insect poison must be constantly on the alert and ready to act fast by administering adrenaline (epinephrine) and consulting a physician. In the US fifty deaths occur each year due to insect stings with many more deaths going unreported.

During the hot summer of 1994 in Germany, bees and wasps swooped down on people for no reason. Page 100 describes in detail how to cope with insect poison allergies. One home remedy for driving off bees and wasps is worth mentioning: Lemon peel stuck with cloves usually keeps the critters at a distance of one meter (Fig. 13). In case you do get stung, however, it often helps to rub the affected area with a peeled onion or alcoholic liniment. The sting or tail should be removed quickly by scratching it with your fingernail. Be careful not to squeeze the area because this will simply release the poison from the poison sac. In order to reduce extreme swelling, doctors can prescribe cortisone which has a general anti-inflammatory effect.

According to a newspaper report, a pilot was said to have mysteriously crashed his plane in Lake Constance for no known reason: all technical errors were ruled out. An autopsy revealed that death was caused by anaphylactic shock, and when his medical history was investigated, it was discovered that he was allergic to insect poison. He had suffered anaphylactic shock when he was stung by a bee trapped in the cockpit, and as he had no emergency equipment with him like an easy-to-use auto-injector, his circulatory system collapsed and he died.

At the back of the book there's a list of what sufferers from insect poison allergy can do to protect themselves and avoid getting stung. Luckily, however, not many allergies have such dramatic, life-threatening consequences.

In order to produce preparations used in the diagnosis and therapy of such allergies, we need a certain quantity of such insect poisons. Bee poison, for example, is produced by stimulating the bee via a weak electric shock to "sting" through a membrane and release its poison (the bee itself is not harmed in the process). The poison is then gathered up and after cleaning – that is, after extraneous proteins have been removed – is used to produce an extract. Producing wasp poison is somewhat more complicated because the sting has to be removed together with the poison. To this end, the wasp is first frozen with the help of liquid nitrogen so that the operation can be carried out under the microscope. Obviously, such an effort makes the poisons expensive. Thus, 1 g of bee poison costs about US $5000 and 1 g of wasp poison up to US $15,000. For this reason, work is now underway to produce the most important allergen of bee poison (phospholipase A2, to which most persons allergic to bee stings react; see the section on the main allergens on pp. 30) by genetic engineering (now I've gone and mentioned it, but only briefly). Through genetic engineering large quantities of substances of very uniform and constant quality can be produced. I shall surely be sitting in my rocking chair before any of these things become standard for human treatment, since the legal and safety hurdles to be crossed before any substance can be used in humans are very high – and rightly so, I think. Many years will pass before all conditions have been fulfilled, but I am confident that such preparations are on the horizon: Genetic engineering has become a very advanced technique.

Finally, a note on the honey bee, so that you can see just how busy these bees really are: In order to produce 1 quart of honey, a bee

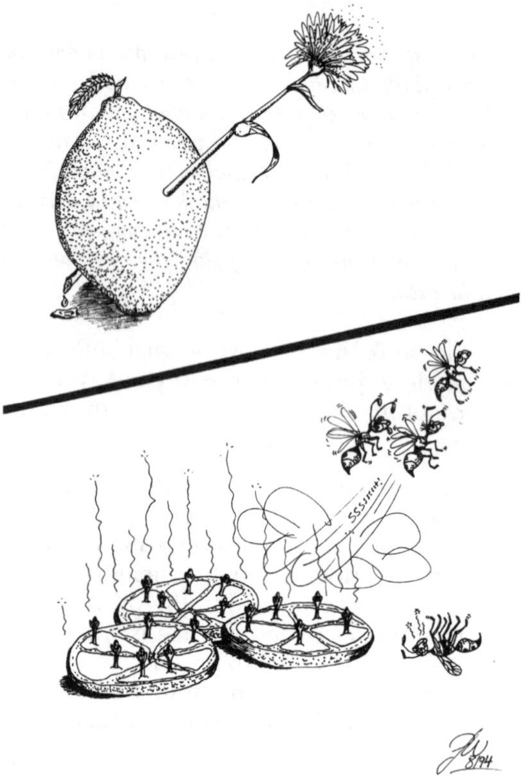

Figure 13: Methods for protecting yourself from bees and wasps: above, wrong; below, right. "Let's get out of here, guys!"

must visit about 10,000,000 blossoms. Honey, too, by the way, can produce allergies (see p. 74).

I'm even allergic to the sun

Who performed "Lazin' on a sunny afternoon in summertime" or "Here comes the sun king" or "Here comes the sun" or "Summer in the city"? It's always the sun (The Stranglers, sounds a bit like Lou Reed), Tequila sunrise (the favorite drink of the Rolling Stones – but what are the aftereffects?). Who sang "I'll follow the sun"? What are the (after) effects of a Tequilla Sunrise? Songs about the sun all express something beautiful, clear (like tequila?) and joyful, but certain predisposed patients can suffer allergic responses to the sun (Fig. 14). There *is* such a thing as a sun allergy. Most of us, myself

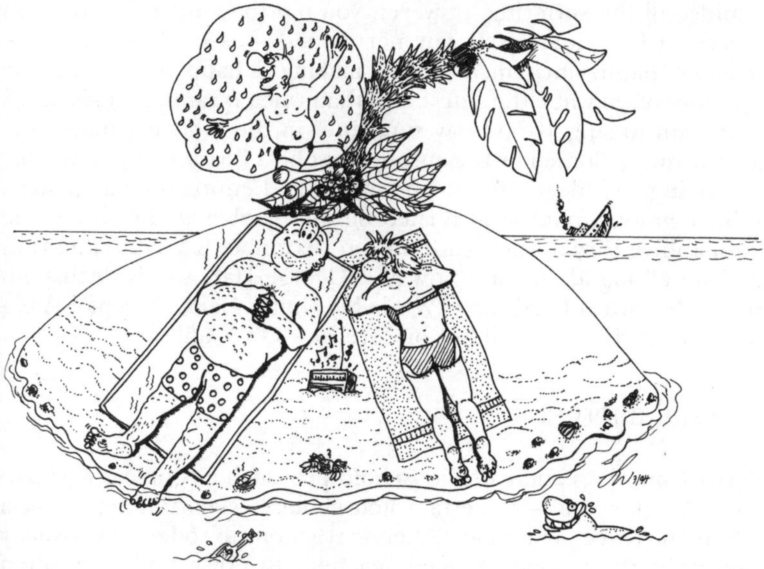

Figure 14. What do I care about red spots and blisters when I can be dreaming of "dancing in the rain." It's all down to what you make of it (he can talk).

included, tend to be more allergic to rain, and those of us who have both the time and the money escape into the sun whenever possible. There is also such a thing as an allergic reaction to cold, but that has been researched even less than the sun. So, what can cause an allergic response to the sun? Usually a combination of suntan lotion (tanning oil), seawater and solar radiation. Allergic reactions connected with suntan lotion could be called "Miami acne" in the United States, since in Europe they are often called "Majorca acne" (Majorca is a very popular holiday island in the Mediterranean off the coast of Spain). Allergy sufferers should therefore discuss their choice of tanning lotion with their dermatologist. After exposure to seawater, they should immediately shower, cover themselves up, and get out of the sun, although some people, strangely, even suffer from sun allergies in the shade. The best thing to do is to avoid the sun altogether. After consulting a doctor, preventive measures can be taken such as swallowing calcium tablets before the trip and packing anti-histamine and possibly cortisone creme in your luggage. Red spots, tiny blisters and extreme itching are the first signs of a sun allergy, and mean it's time to change lotions and avoid the sun. Oil of St. John's Wort is an all natural miracle cure which soothes the affected area and reduces itching. Because the skin is so thin, the forehead is one of the most sensitive spots for developing a sun allergy.

Amidst all the suffering, however, you mustn't forget that the sun makes us feel vital, calms our nerves and – as my brother says – releases "happy hormones," simply making us happier. People smile far more often when the sun shines than when it rains, and it's much more fun to sing "Good day sunshine" in the morning than "Rai-ai-ai-ai-ain." ("Somehow the author must be a Beatles fan," you must be saying – indeed he is, and of John Lennon in particular). John Lennon would have turned 60 on October 9, 2000, and the 20th anniversary of this death was on December 8, 2000. Time flies and we all tag along, and now also George Harrison is dead – no more "My Sweet Lord" and "While My Guitar Gently Weeps"? A big loss. But their songs will live on forever – Oh Yeah!!

Animal allergens

Apart from dogs and cats, household pets such as guinea pigs, parrots, hamsters and – in certain households – even rats represent a potential source of allergies. Allergic reactions to rodents are usually caused by their urine, whereas reactions to down quilts are often caused by duck, goose, and chicken feathers – or even storage mites. The same is true for parrots and other exotic birds although bird lime on the feathers can sometimes cause the allergies as well. But as the following example shows, what you thought was an allergic reaction to an animal can be something else entirely.

A patient thought she was allergic to her parrot, yet the in vivo tests all came back negative. When the search for the allergen was continued in true Sherlock Holmes style, the culprit was discovered in the sunflower seeds she fed the parrot. So don't omit the animal's food as a potential source of allergies!

People with an aquarium are thus less likely to be allergic to their live pets ("A Fish Called Wanda") than to what they feed them, e. g., water fleas.

Zookeepers can sensitize themselves to monkey urine, elephant hair and low-bellied pig hair, but as most of us rarely keep such animals as pets, there is little risk of the average pet-owner sensitizing him or herself. People allergic to cat hair, however, can even register a response to the lion act at the circus.

The following case – almost worthy of an Agatha Christie plot – demonstrates how aggressive animal hair can be:

About 17 years ago a woman's body was found in a forest near the German city of Frankfurt. Foul play was suspected, but there was no evidence of violence. Upon rigorously checking the victim's medical history, it was found that she was allergic to horsehair. So it was deduced that while she was walking in the woods, allergens inhaled from horses riding by had induced anaphylactic shock, from which she died.

Luckily for us, animal allergies only very rarely take such a dramatic turn. In most cases, animals are a source of pleasure and improve our quality of life. To avoid sensitization, however, it is advisable not to have animals in the house for the first 3–5 months of a baby's life. But in 2005 the opposite advice will probably be given! As Bob Dylan sings "The times they are a changing." Why not in allergy research, too?

Plants and your apartment

House dust and all its components have already been discussed (p. 18), but what about plants (excluding carnivorous ones) in your apartment?

A patient complained again and again about how he felt at the office. (Such complaints are not necessarily confined to allergies, of course). House dust mites and animal hair tests were carried out, but both proved negative. When questioned by his doctor, the patient recalled the Ficus benjamina plant in his office. The office dust was inspected and found to contain large amounts of plant allergen. Skin tests made with extracts from the leaves and stem showed positive, indicating the patient was allergic to that particular house plant. A RAST of the patient's serum ascertained the presence of the relevant IgE as well.

In many homes, *Ficus benjamina* ("weeping fig," see Fig. 15) has almost completely replaced the good old rubber plant. My mother used to rub the leaves of her rubber tree with beer to make them shiny; a *Ficus benjamina* could take a whole case – what a waste!

But how is it possible to be allergic to *Ficus benjamina* leaves if you don't touch them? The answer is that the leaves secrete a latex-like fluid (here we go again with latex) which combines with house dust and, when blown through the air, is distributed around the apartment and finally inhaled by the patient, causing an allergic reaction.

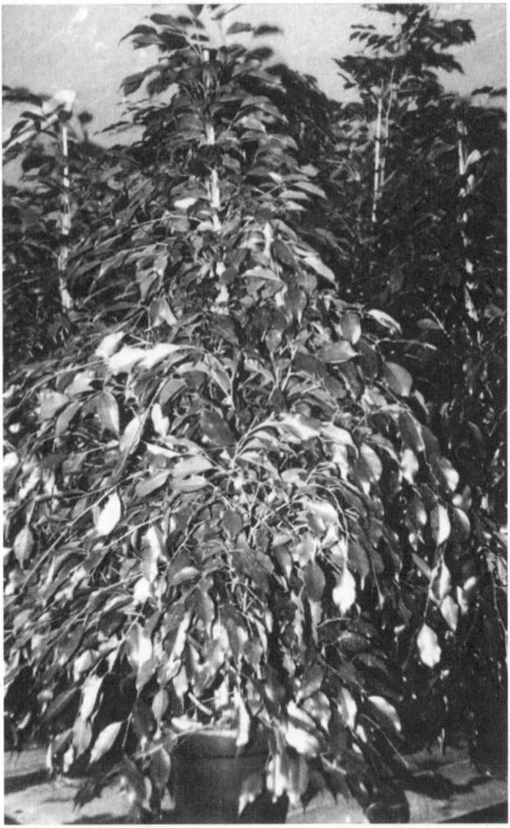

Figure 15. Ficus benjamina in my home.

Ficus benjamina plants are frequently to be found in hospital lobbies and asthma clinics, a fact which could (and should) quickly be altered after reading this passage. It may even signify the return of the good old rubber plant which so happily crawled along the ceilings in homes all over the Western world.

Who can be affected by allergies?

Can anyone be affected by pollen, house dust mites, animal hair and insect poison? Scientific studies show that certain factors determine when and if an individual is allergy prone.

One thing is certain: allergies are mainly inherited. People with an inherited predisposition are called atopic. The approximate risk for a newborn baby is 50–70% if both parents suffer the same allergic symptoms. This risk only decreases slightly (40–60%) if both parents have allergies but different symptoms. If only one parent or sibling is allergic, the risk decreases further to 20–40%. However, even if no member of the family is allergic, a newborn infant still has a 5–15% chance of developing allergies.

Non-atopic people themselves are not totally spared and can sensitize themselves to particularly aggressive substances in the course of their work.

Here's an interesting case for all you twins researchers. My wife, Irene, and her sister, Evi, are monozygotic twins, born some 15 minutes apart. Evi developed at age 50 a severe hay fever. She is not a typical atopic person. My wife, on the other hand, has no allergic reactions, save for a very slight reaction to mugwort. Whatever else may be true about identical twins, it's not the case for allergies. This example also shows that it is possible to become suddenly afflicted by allergies even at a later point in life. Evi has a clear allergic reaction to the pollen of hazel nut, birch and alder trees. She is considering an immunotherapy to avoid the allergy from spreading to the lower respiratory tracts. She started hyposensitization, but because she is also plagued by rheumatism, she had to break it off due to the severe side effects. The quiz question for the medical colleagues reading this: Is rheumatism a contraindication to hyposensitization?

Some people involved in the coffee industry who work with the unroasted coffee-bean, have suffered watering eyes and runny noses due to constant contact with aggressive allergens. Have no fear, you cannot sensitize yourself to roasted coffee, only unroasted coffee beans are allergenic: the roasting process destroys the allergens and with them any risk of sensitization. In a worker in a factory where coffee beans are roasted we found an allergy to roasted coffee. In further serological tests we discovered that there were differences even in his reactions to various brands of coffee. I should note, however, that allergy to roasted coffee is and remains very very rare.

A more interesting discovery was that some of the dockworkers had an allergic reaction to castor beans. What's the story here? Investigations showed that not only coffee beans, but also ground castor beans were being shipped in the same bags. The bags themselves had thus been polluted with castor-oil. Since castor-oil is a very potent allergen, the dockworkers had become sensitized to it and eventually had allergic reactions. This particularly well-hidden allergen could be found out only after intensive contact with the persons concerned.

Why do more and more people suffer from allergies? The latest theories

The increasing number of allergy sufferers is often put down to the increase in environmental pollution, so: Get rid of cars! No more industry! Close the power plants! For a long time, this argument was considered valid, but now, very different reasons are being discussed. By improving the insulation in our apartments and leaving no cracks for the dampness to escape, we create ideal conditions for house dust mites. In increasing our standards of personal hygiene and showering several times a day, we destroy our natural skin oils, rendering our bodies more susceptible to allergens.

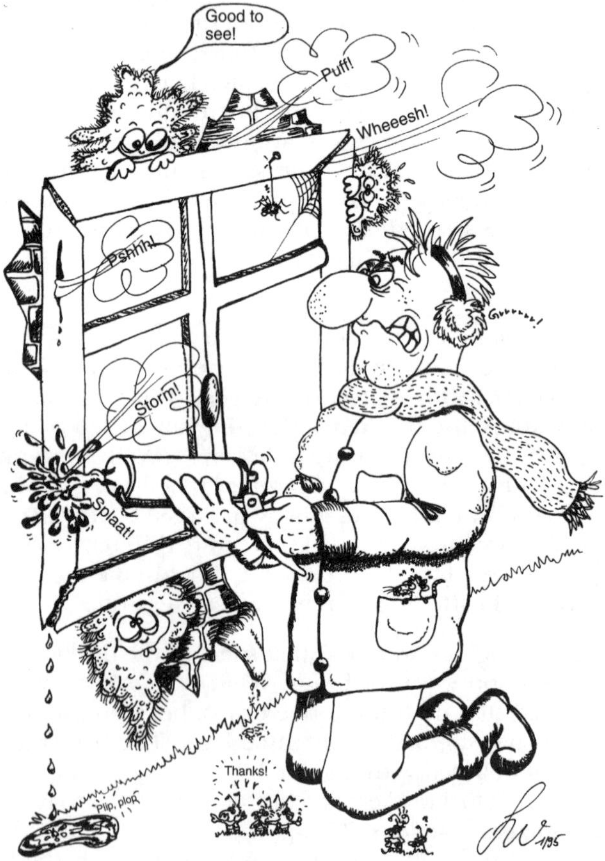

Figure 16. Support your local mites and mold and pick up that silicone gun!

House pets play a major role as well. In Germany, for instance, 40% of households keep pets, and every third household has a cat, making for a total of around 5.5 million feline pets. Around 40% of UK households also keep pets, and cat will be present in 60% of these households. It seems that in the Western world we simply invite the allergens into our homes! Another development which encourages both house dust mites and mold to settle into our homes is modern glazing which – thanks to the silicone seal – is far less permeable than previous fenestration (see Fig. 16), allowing almost no circulation of air. In Denmark they anticipated the dangers of excessive home insulation, and built gaps into the walls of their houses with screens to keep out insects and to provide the necessary ventilation. In case you're planning to build a house, don't forget that adequate air circulation reduces the risk of allergies and gives you plenty of fresh air!

Another theory suggests that our immune system is in fact bored, and rather than sit around twiddling its thumbs, it becomes overly active. The boredom is caused by a lack of real enemies such as worms or parasites, so it now treats pollen and house dust mites as such. The theory is quite attractive and will no doubt be further pursued, undergoing far more investigation before it can be proven valid, but let's hope that in the meantime our immune systems don't die of boredom and fight against the substances which make up our own bodies!

Newer theories – the city/country phenomenon

Have any newer theories cropped up to explain this state of affairs? The clear answer to this question is yes – something we can attribute to the keen observations of a Swiss country doctor.

During his work with people who live in the country, away from the cities, he noticed fewer allergies than among the city folks (see Fig. 17). Apparently people living in the country have more direct contact with animal epithelia, mold, mites, and pollen – but strangely enough have overall fewer allergic reactions. Perhaps the reason lies in their living more in contact and harmony with nature; maybe they ate (literally) more dirt as children, not only without dying from it, but actually strengthening their immune system to boot. Eating dirt can help the immune system by having it react to the "contaminants" in the dirt – the true enemies of humankind – and not against such pseudo-enemies as pollen. This should not be taken to say that we should all enjoy a tablespoon full of dirt with our morning cornflakes; rather it is meant to show that supposed dangers (children playing

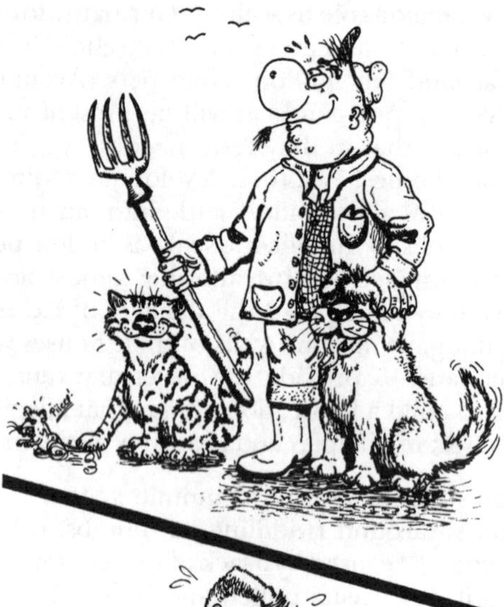

Figure 17: Better a free-breathing country bumpkin than a runny-nosed, stressed-out yuppie.

in the dirt, puddles, etc.) sometimes aren't. Where can a child play in a puddle these days in the big city (especially without being scrubbed off afterwards with soap and disinfectant!)? Maybe it's not so bad after all to live in harmony with nature and come to terms with natural things, like bacteria, and not to avoid them at all costs. Think about our mouthsprays, lozenges, gargling solutions, etc., with their "antibacterial effects." Today, we even have antibacterial jogging socks, true to the motto: Don't give nature a chance!

There was once a Woody Allen movie ("The Sleeper," if I'm not mistaken) where he made fun of everything that in 1970 was held to be bad for your health by having it held in 2170 as being good for your health. Sometimes that's the way I see the present-day discussion surrounding allergies.

A professor once put it very succinctly during a meeting: Low income, poor hygiene, poor education and a home in the country – that's what keeps you from getting allergies. That may be an exaggeration, but not much of one. The Swiss country doctor certainly had no idea of the importance his observations would have one day.

(A side note for the scientists and doctors among my readers: The endotoxins play a major role in this country/city phenomenon, something supported especially by recent studies.)

This question promises to be remain an interesting and exciting one in the future.

Does having siblings decrease the risk of allergies? Another theory

Not only is having brothers and sisters much more fun than being a single child (I've got two) but according to the latest studies, it makes you less prone to allergies. How can this be explained? Children who have siblings come into closer contact with infectious diseases such as worm infestation, measles, and German measles, which (according to studies carried out in the Czech Republic and West Germany) are thought possibly to protect against allergies. Although air pollution in the Czech Republic is far higher than in West Germany, more allergy sufferers were found in the cleaner west than in the highly polluted areas of the Czech Republic. One explanation for this lies in the fact that the people of those regions live closer together and in much larger families than in Germany, resulting in a greater risk of infection but possibly a reduced susceptibility to allergies. It can also be assumed that these people's immune systems don't waste their time fighting amiable allergens such as pollen and house dust mites, preferring to concentrate on the real enemy. The theory is still quite recent but nonetheless fascinating, and will certainly invite further research. So let's "come together ... right now!" and prevent allergies as well!

Allergies and cancer – and something else of interest

Our immune system plays an important role in diseases such as allergies and cancer. An allergologist friend of mine told me that in his 24 years of experience, not one of the allergy patients he treated had cancer. How can that be explained? One thing allergies do is challenge our immune system and provoke it, causing it to react. Thus it has been suggested that one possible "side-effect" of this process is a protection against the growth of tumors. Results from a study done at the University Clinic in Göttingen, Germany, show allergy sufferers have a 50% lower risk of contracting melanosis. In Holland, medical experts have similarly proven that allergies can provide protection against cancer of the pancreas.

Here too, research has only just begun. If protection against cancer turned out to be a positive side effect of having allergies, allergy patients would perhaps not suffer quite so much. Here we have another field open for interdisciplinary study.

Songs against allergies?

Although there have been vague attempts at connecting tinnitus (a sound in the ear) – a disease from which more and more people suffer – with allergic reactions, and music therapy (Mozart's violin concertos via headphones) has eased the suffering of several tinnitus patients, there is no evidence that music therapy can help allergy sufferers. But in spite of the doubts a "little light music" here may help you to relax (see Fig. 18).

1

Allergic People

Text and Music: Rüdiger Wahl
Arrangement: Werner Lang

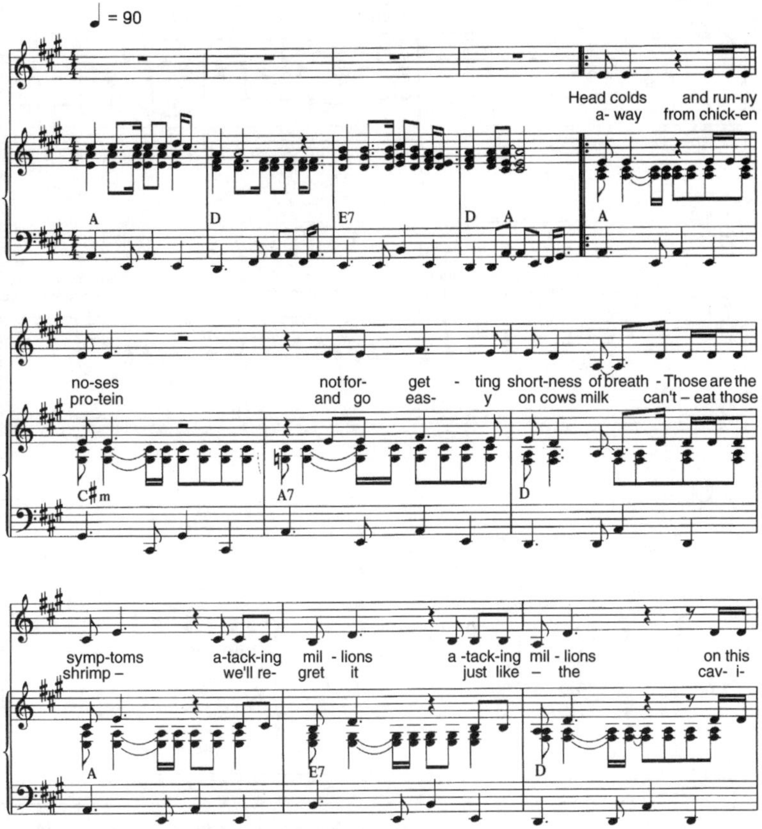

Figure 18. And yet another song: "Allergic People." ©MCA Music GmbH, Hamburg für die Welt

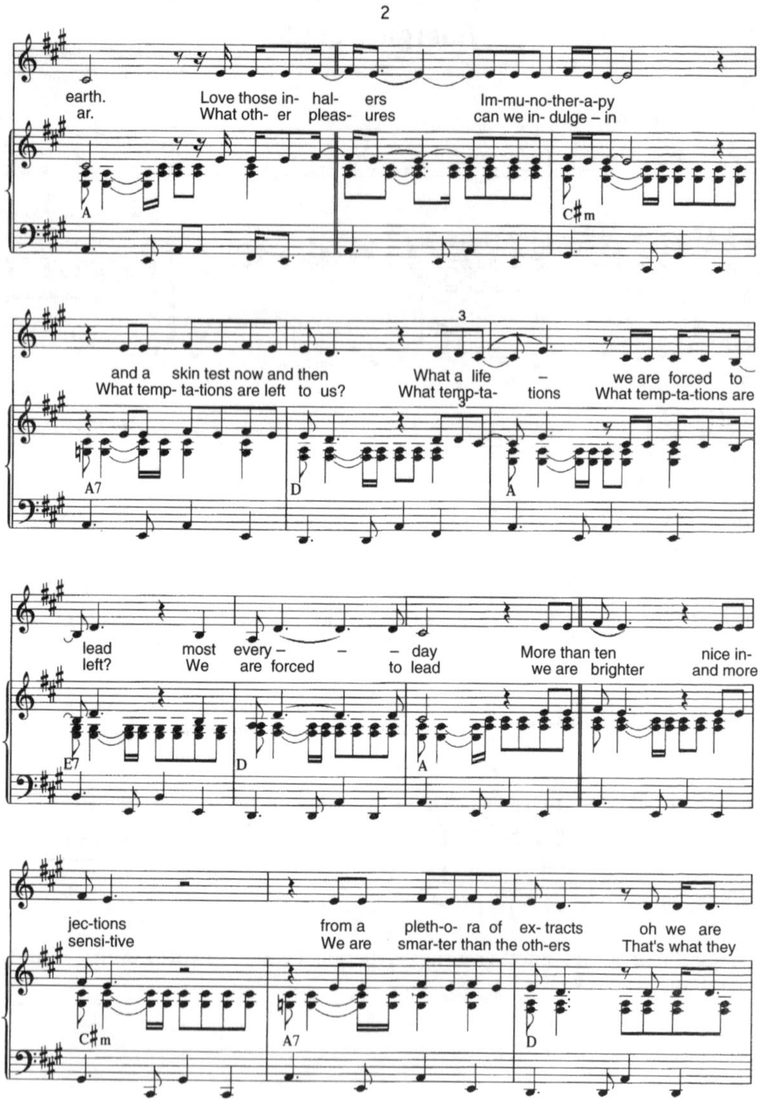

Figure 18. "Allergic People" (continued)

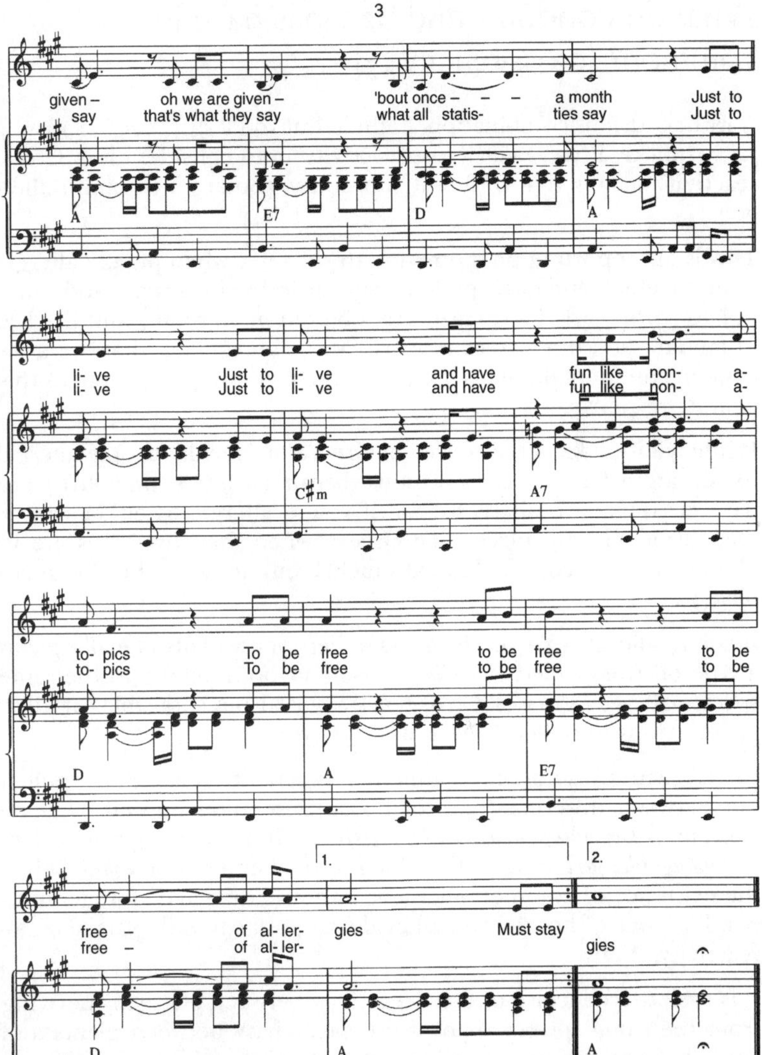

Figure 18. "Allergic People" (continued)

What do condoms and bananas have in common? (cross-reactivity)

A rather curious combination, I admit, but you'll discover the answer fairly quickly if you take "cross-reactivity" into consideration. Cross-reactivity means that different substances contain a common allergen.

This is an important phenomenon to consider when people allergic to birch, alder, and hazel pollen begin suffering in January and again in late April/early May. Hazel trees bloom in Germany and the UK in January and birch trees in April/May, and the fact that the trees contain common allergens, i. e., cross-reactive allergens, explains this allergic response.

While lying under an olive tree in Greece or Florida, people allergic to ash can suffer an allergic response because ash trees and olive trees have cross-reactive allergens. So, if you're allergic to either ash or lilac, avoid visiting places like Greece when the olive trees are in bloom! As a Grecophile I'm extremely thankful not to be allergic to olive trees!

If you're allergic to Timothy grass pollen, you will also be allergic to a type of grass called *Dactylis glomerata* as both belong to the same species of sweet grasses. Cross-reactivity is also responsible for allergic reactions to pollen from grass and rye.

Cross-reactivity is not only common between different types of pollen but between different types of house dust mites as well. Anyone allergic to *Dermatophagoides pteronyssinus* will also be allergic to *Dermatophagoides farinae* as both belong to the family *Pyroglyphid*. While the existence of common allergens in house dust and storage mites is still a topic of hot debate, all evidence points to only partial cross-reactivity, if any.

It is easier to conceive of cross-reactivity between allergens deriving from the same species than of cross-reactivity between plants and animals from different species, but as hard as this is to explain, it exists.

A patient allergic to birch pollen suffered a serious allergic reaction to Granny Smith and Golden Delicious apples (both of which look better than they taste). This response was caused by the cross-reactive allergens in birch trees and apples.

Not only with respect to this volume has much changed since 1993, apple fashions have changed, too. I don't see as many sorts of green apples displayed today in the stores. Rather, they tend to be red or yellow (there's yellow again), with names such as Royal Gala, Braeburn – and they taste good. I still eat an apple every day, for in my opinion the saying is still true: An apple a day keeps the doctor away. (My doctor readers may forgive me.) However, I don't have any information as such on the allergenicity of the newer apple types. The following three varieties are listed in order of their allergenicity: Golden Delicious, Granny Smith, and Jonagold. Gloster, Hammerstein, and Jamba (an old German variety my grandmother Paula had in her garden), in that order, are easier for allergy sufferers to tolerate. The allergenicity of apples has also been linked to their degree of ripeness. Unripe apples are less allergenic than ripe ones, but in addition to tasting inferior, they can also cause digestive problems.

Figure 19 illustrates further foods associated with birch pollen allergy: tomatoes (raw), potatoes (raw), apples, peaches, apricots, cherries, almonds, celery (raw), carrots (raw), alder, hazel and hazelnut.

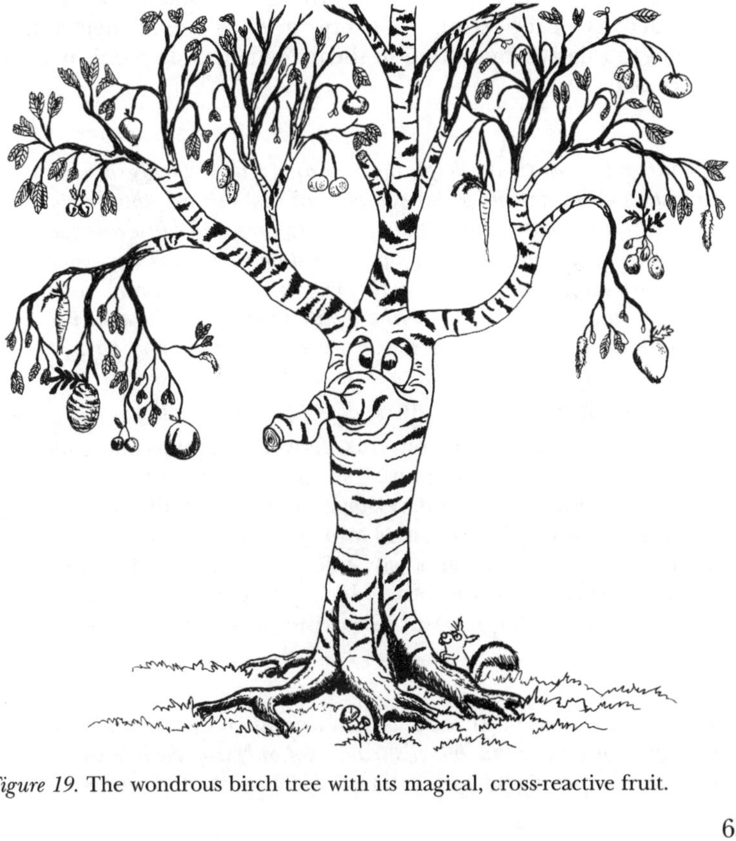

Figure 19. The wondrous birch tree with its magical, cross-reactive fruit.

Celery, onions and garlic can also cause allergies in people allergic to **mugwort** due to the cross-reactive allergens.

One new point of discussion is the partial allergic cross-reaction between the house dust mite and crustaceans such as crabs, shrimps, and lobsters. This is an amazing thing. Studies show that they have a common allergen, the tropomyosin, which is also found in the common housefly. The latter may thus one day also have a partial cross-reaction with the house dust mite because of the common substance, tropomyosin. This is an example of how we are always looking for the common ground of the various "stuffs"of allergy in order to prove scientifically cross-reactivity.

A further cross-reactivity may be found between mugwort pollen, carrots, celery and lychee – that slippery fruit that plops out of the mouth when you try to eat it.

The common protein is profilin. It would take several chapters to do justice to substances such as profilin and tropomyosin, but that is not my topic here. Suffice it to say that the commonalities behind the cross-reactivity of the "stuffs" of allergy are not due to their botanic or zoological classes, but rather to the protein and allergenic patterns they contain.

A fruit grower who was allergic to house dust mite suddenly suffered an asthma attack while picking apples. At first this was thought to have been caused by overexertion, which is known to cause allergic reactions in athletes (exercise-induced asthma). But as her work wasn't very strenuous, this possibility was discarded. Examinations and laboratory tests revealed that the patient was allergic to the red spider mite in the apple tree. Upon further investigation, partial cross-reactivity was discovered to exist between the house dust mite Dermatophagoides pteronyssinus and the red spider mite.

Now let us return to that curious link between bananas and condoms. Condoms, balloons, rubber gloves, surgical gloves, rubberbands, the sticky side of Band-Aids and postage stamp glue all contain latex. Studies have shown that bananas and latex have cross-reactive allergens (Fig. 20), which explains why many people who are allergic to one are also allergic to the other. In my case, only banana peel underfoot produces allergic responses from my immune system.

While on vacation in Africa a woman was bitten by a monkey (as strange as it may sound, but it's true). Not only was the bite painful, she subsequently suffered an anaphylactic shock. At the hospital it was discovered that she had an allergy to latex. The solution to this puzzle? Before biting the woman the monkey had eaten a banana and thus had passed on this substance to her. Because of the cross-reactivity of banana and latex, the woman suffered a severe allergic reaction.

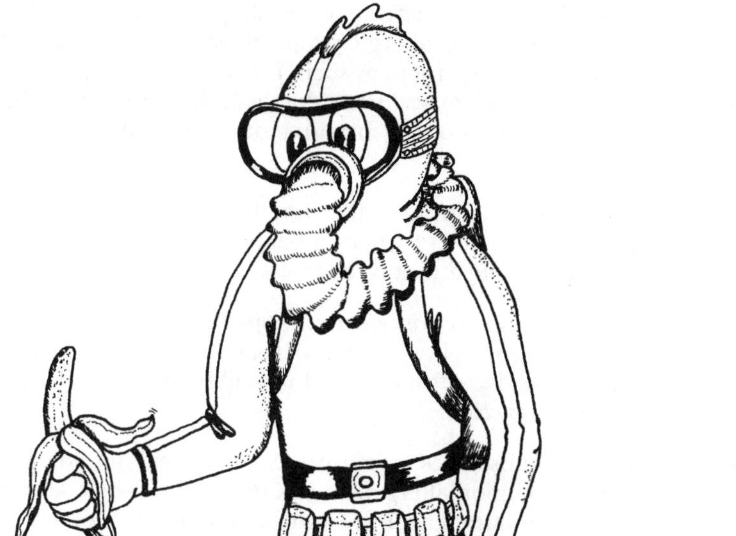

Figure 20. How not to dress and what not to eat if you're allergic to latex!

This is an example of how very careful allergic persons must be. This particular case was so interesting and so unusual that it eventually made its way into a scientific journal.

More and more people are developing latex allergies and it appears to be *the* allergen of today as well as tomorrow. French studies have shown that 34% of atopic individuals (see p. 54) can show reactions to latex. In spina bifida patients, that is, in children with an exposed spinal cord, who are often operated on and thus have frequent contact with the latex in OR gloves, the rate of sensitization to latex lies around 40% to 50%. Latex is definitely the allergen of our time. Since the allergen is so aggressive, allergic people must always wear a necklace or bracelet identifying them as such. If emergency surgery must be performed (e. g., after an accident), doctors will be warned against wearing latex gloves and possibly bringing on an anaphylactic shock during the operation.

Latex allergens are so aggressive that one highly sensitized patient had only to enter a beer tent where a balloon was attached to the ceiling to suffer an acute attack of asthma.

That was a short digression on latex, a subject deserving of at least a chapter if not an entire book. Let's wait and see what the future will bring regarding this substance and its ability to cause allergies. Now back to cross-reactivity.

Just how it is that substances from different botanical or zoological species can have common allergens is still unknown. People allergic to pollen should be warned against eating certain foods which could cause a pollen-associated cross-reactive food allergy. I have included a chart of cross-reactive substances at the back of this book.

When considering cross-reactivity, however, it must be remembered that independent sensitization is also possible. If a person reacts to both grass pollen and mold, such as *Alternaria tenuis* or *Penicillium notatum*, for example, this is due to independent sensitization rather than a cross-reactivity. Today we have a variety of chemical immunity methods for scientifically proving the cross-reactivity of substances.

Whether there is a cross-reactivity between drinking Bavarian beer and eating a Bavarian *wurst* may be doubted – although this suspicion was once aired (perhaps an April Fools' joke?). One patient evidenced allergic reactions after consuming a meal of Bavarian beer and *wurst*. (What the relevant article did not mention, however, was exactly how many beers had to be consumed to produce this reaction.) Nevertheless, some people do have allergic reactions to beer or wine because of the ingredients such as yeast, the yeast-like fungus *Candida albicans*, malt, sulfites (a pseudoallergen), etc., but rarely to the alcohol itself. Reactions to *wurst* – whatever its origin – are usually to the spices contained therein.

A recent case was described of an allergic reaction to wurst where the source was ascorbic acid (vit. C), which had been added to the product. An example of a further allergen gone undeclared on the package.

Allergy to food substances

Allergies to foodstuffs are often discussed with great fervor, and we would like to take the tone down a notch. Every human being consumes up to the age of 70 a total of some 52 tons of food. A normal visit to the local supermarket with a full shopping cart means taking home somewhere between 6,000 and 8,000 different substances – proteins, carbohydrates, preservatives, etc. And, yet, despite the breadth and amount of foodstuffs we intake, allergies to foods are by far not the most common ones found. With respect to the total population in Germany, for example, the percentage of food allergies in children lies at about 2% to 7%, in adults at about 2% to 4%. Subjectively, up to 18% to 20% of all adults *think* they have (or have experienced) a food allergy. Often, however, it is not a true allergy, but rather an incompatibility with some component of a meal. Pseudo-allergies (see also p. 5) caused by preservatives lie at around 0.9%.

Obviously, the attention given in the media to food allergies is highly exaggerated, which is not say that there are not severely allergenic foods out there, such as peanuts or kiwis. Let us look at a few food allergies in more detail.

Why can't I eat eggs?

Food allergies are becoming more and more common (but see my relativization above). The United States Department of Agriculture estimates that some 34 million adults and children are allergic to some food products. Estimates of cow's milk allergy are reported to range from 0.3 to 7.7% of the population. But the incidence is higher in infants than in adults.

One reason for the increase of food allergies could be that many varieties of fruit are available today, all year round. Another reason might be that meat and sandwich meats are now often seasoned, and bread is rarely available in pure form without the addition of nuts, linseed, or sunflower seeds. Recently I even saw an advertisement for pumpkin seed bread. What next, appleseed and cherry stone varieties? Modern man is bombarded from all sides with so many kinds of foods and preservatives, it's no wonder he becomes sensitized, especially if atopic.

Egg and milk allergies are at the very top of the food allergy hit list. These allergies often appear in infant years, usually going away later in life, but an effective way to prevent their presence in the first place is to breastfeed as long as possible, and afterwards to feed the baby hypoallergenic food. Since such food sometimes still contains ever so slight allergenic traces, those children acutely allergic to cows' milk should be given a skin or serum test by their doctor. Hypoallergenic food is not only suitable as a milk substitute but can be used in preparing delicious meals. There are even cookbooks available.

In addition to milk and eggs, the most common sources of food allergies include shrimp, lobster, prawns, mussels, and fish; flour such as rye and wheat; and spices and nuts, particularly peanuts and hazelnuts. Raw potatoes can also cause allergies when you peel them.

A doctor once asked me to test the serum of a patient for a Beluga caviar allergy (the patient wasn't Joan Collins, funnily enough). What a tragic loss in the quality of everyday life that could be – no more Beluga caviar – perish the thought! The doctor sent us a small jar of the alleged allergen and after testing several milligrams, the rest was dispatched with a bottle of champagne. (How we love our work sometimes!) Our tests showed no trace of allergies and we passed the good news on to the doctor, no doubt to the immense relief of the poor patient. But it must be added that seafood is a high risk allergen for people with a corresponding predisposition.

Although rice is eaten by millions of people every day, there is very little international documentation of rice allergies.

We discovered a rice allergy in a patient which occurred whilst at a wedding, when she took a handful of rice to throw at the bride and groom. A form of urticaria broke out on the backs of her hands. After eating cooked rice, she showed food allergy symptoms, which included not only indigestion but also a runny nose and asthma.

Another food allergy not to be ignored is what I call "Chinese Restaurant Syndrome" in which a patient can suffer hot flushes and even have difficulty breathing. This is caused by the numerous spices used in Chinese cooking as well as flavor enhancers such as monosodium glutamate (MSG). I am lucky in that my favorite cuisine is Italian and I've yet to hear of someone being allergic to spaghetti! Very aggressive is peanut. Many food allergic people in the United States show allergic reactions to peanut. Some airlines have even stopped offering passengers food that contains peanuts – to protect them from possible reactions.

Often what appears at first to be a food allergy in the end reveals itself to be only an intolerance. This can be determined by an oral provocation test (see p. 87) administered by a doctor.

Artificial coloring and preservatives can also play a major role in causing allergies. One of the most common allergenic coloring agents is tartrazine, which was formerly used in red and yellow gummybears (type of gumdrop). But is it really always the coloring agent?

In the middle of the night – why, I do not know – a patient consumed several handfuls of gummybears, suffered anaphylactic shock and had to be taken to the hospital. Luckily she was soon out of danger, and the search for the allergen began. Tartrazine was naturally considered first, but when her doctor administered an oral test of several milligrams, nothing happened. Further enquiries revealed that gummybears also contain gelatine, and sure enough, laboratory tests showed a very strong reaction to the substance. Studies on cross-reactivity showed that plasma volume expanders contain modified gelatine and they must be avoided when treating people allergic to gelatine.

Although gelatine is used in countless candy items such as marshmallows ("... eating marshmallow pie ..." – who sang that?) and is often added to yogurt, very little has been documented concerning gelatine allergies and we can assume that the substance is not highly allergenic. When investigating the causes of allergic reactions to candy items, however, it is important to remember that gelatine *can* cause an allergic response. With allergic reactions to vaccinations one should always consider the gelatine or modified gelatine present in some vaccines.

Today, tartrazine in gummybears is no longer an issue since fruit juices are used as a coloring agent, making the candy – in my opinion – not nearly as good a chew, but far, far better for you.

When a food allergy is presumed but provocation or serum tests fail to show positive, additives such as preservatives and coloring (used to stabilize and "improve" foods) should always be taken into consideration. People allergic to acetylsalicylic acid (aspirin) should know, for instance, that many foods including even some fruit contain salicylic acid, and must be avoided. In many countries, sadly, there is as yet no legislation compelling manufacturers to furnish a detailed list of all ingredients in foods and cosmetics: such a law would make it far easier to determine what substances cause the allergic reaction. For example, a patient had an allergic reaction to shaving creme, and after lengthy investigation, green peppers were found to be the culprit. Who on earth would have suspected green peppers to be used in the manufacture of shaving creme, even if the can was bright green?

The opening of the borders in Europe has led to even more exotic foods entering the country, and of course further allergens as well. Think of the traces of animal hairs found in cookies.

And what of food allergies abroad, the foods you normally don't eat at home? Let's take Greece as an example. . .

In June 1994, my wife and I spent our summer vacation on the Greek island of Crete. After nearly every meal (which I must say I really enjoyed: tsatziki and real, sun-soaked tomatoes, not the ones they grow on straw) my wife complained of nausea and indigestion which gave her diarrhea and made her vomit. I recalled that she had complained similarly six months before after eating Greek food back home in Hamburg, Germany. Such symptoms can be caused by a food allergy, and I suspected a spice allergy, for, as every Grecophile knows, Greek food is seasoned with various local spices. My wife's discomfort was unfortunately so acute that we had to cut short our vacation and fly home, where we now intend to have in vitro and in vivo tests carried out by an allergologist. These tests could prove difficult, however, as many spices used in Greece are not available in Germany. Further- more, dried herbs and spices are usually used for test extracts in Germany whereas the ones used in Greece are usually fresh, and this could possibly affect the allergen pattern. Nonetheless, we will certainly carry out these tests, which I sincerely hope will prove negative, otherwise: Goodbye Greece! The suburbs of Hamburg are nice and green, but don't offer quite as much in the way of sun and sea ... At least we wouldn't have any trouble with the language.

P. S. The *in vitro* test for mugwort pollen came back positive, which means that my suspicions of a spice allergy weren't so far off, as mugwort and spices are cross-reactive (see p. 64).

Allergic to alcohol?

Allergic reactions to the alcohol contained in alcoholic beverages are to my knowledge unknown. There are, however, documented cases of allergic reactions after consumption of alcoholic beverages. The decisive things are the substances contained in the drinks.

After a glass of Campari a woman suffered a severe allergic reaction and had to be hospitalized. After the symptoms had subsided, Campari was tested in a rub test (see p. 85), and a positive reaction was observed. The search set out for the source, and a red dye (carmin) made from lice bred on cacti on Fuerteventura (Canary Islands) was discovered to be the culprit after direct skin tests. This solved the mystery of her reaction to Campari. A very new remark: Recently it was discovered that it was not in fact the red dye itself, but the animal proteins with which the red dye was contaminated which caused the reaction.

In beer allergy, which definitively does not occur only after the tenth glass (you should be so lucky), the allergenic culprits could be the hops and malt contained.

As to wine, the sulfites are presumably the cause of allergic reactions, stemming from the use of wooden kegs for storage (pseudoallergy).

In any alcohol allergy one must always consider the individual ingredients – or the allergy is being used as an excuse (see Fig. 21).

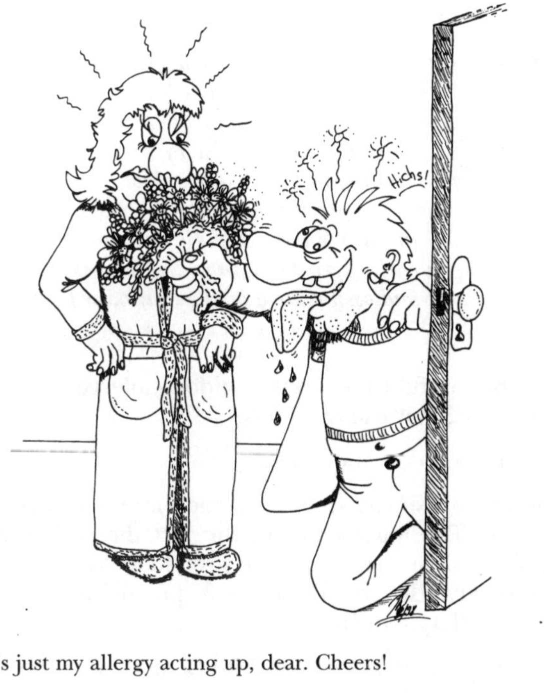

Figure 21. It's just my allergy acting up, dear. Cheers!

Hidden allergens

It's certainly nice to know which pure foods you are allergic to, but hidden allergens make things much more complicated. Is it the nuts in the chocolate, the egg in the cake, the milk in a variety of milk products or the MSG in Chinese food? One important hidden allergen is celery, which is used in a variety of processed foods, fast-food meals, salts, etc., but often not expressly mentioned in the list of ingredients. Because of cross-reactivity, persons allergic to mugwort are at greatest risk. Soy products are also often used anonymously and can be considered a hidden allergen. To discover the hidden allergens you have to go on an "elimination diet" which means eating only potatoes or rice (as long as you are not allergic to them) under close supervision in a hospital. The suspect foods are then inserted into the diet and the allergen is discovered by simple process of elimination. It is there, of course, that the difficulties begin: the patient has to try to avoid such foods, but where can you get cake made without eggs? One side effect of the "elimination diet" is to lose weight – not always a bad thing.

Hidden allergens are sometimes hidden in roundabout ways:

After eating a slice of bread and honey a girl suffered a severe allergic reaction. The flour allergy test came back negative, but that for honey was clearly positive. The ingredient responsible in the honey was unclear. The girl's medical history revealed that she was allergic to mugwort, leading us to the culprit: Honey often contains sunflower pollen and mugwort and sunflower pollen are cross-reactive. In vivo and in vitro tests for allergic reactions to sunflower pollen were consequently carried out and came back positive, proving that the allergy had been caused by the sunflower pollen in the honey.

One should be careful to remember hidden allergens such as pollen when dealing with natural products.

There are other hidden allergens:

People allergic to fish can show a reaction after eating eggs. "*Why?*" might you ask. The answer lies in the fact that chickenfeed often contains fish meal, and traces of fish protein make their way into the egg. These survive the cooking process, provoking an allergic reaction in people allergic to fish.

Recently during a visit to the "Sea Life Center" near the Baltic Sea I learned that fish oil is sometimes put into cookies. This may also be a case of hidden allergen heretofore unknown in the literature.

A woman with a well-known allergic reaction to chicken eggs had a severe reaction to a piece of strawberry candy. The skin-prick test was positive. Further investigation revealed that ovalbumin was being used a thickening agent. Ovalbumin is the major allergen (see p. 30) of the chicken egg. A case for Lieutenant Columbo!

A footnote for my friends from Bremen (Germany): The traditional meal of kale with a particular type of sausage made with beef brain (something I've had to do without in times of BSE) sometimes causes a reaction in persons allergic to nickel because kale has a high concentration of nickel.

Tragic news for those with a nickel allergy: Nickel is to be found in chocolate, along with the milk, cocoa and nuts. If you show an allergic reaction after eating chocolate – spare a penny for the thought that it might be the nickel.

A newly discovered hidden allergen

With hidden allergens one usually first thinks of undeclared substances in processed foods. Here I want to mention an interesting hidden allergen that is not a food additive.

This allergen should be considered in cases where a fish allergy is present. Studies have shown that some patients exhibiting a reaction to raw fish are in fact reacting to a parasite that naturally occurs in all seafood, namely, anisakis. This should be considered when diagnosing such an allergic reaction.

Allergic reactions to anisakis can lead to stomach problems, urticaria, skin reactions, and in rare cases even to anaphylaxis (see p. 1). Thus, we are dealing here with a naturally occurring, albeit hidden allergen.

The exact role of parasites as sources of allergic reactions has not been studied extensively. This study on anisakis is just the beginning.

Genetically engineered foods – a danger for atopic persons?

Recently, some foods have been genetically engineered in order to make plants more resistant to certain pests or pesticides, or in order to increase the overall amount of protein. This can produce cases of hidden allergens that may cause reactions in respective candidates. Finding the culprit can be a difficult matter since nowhere is it mentioned exactly how the food has been genetically modified. Some cases have been described in the literature. For example, one well-known food allergen wound up being transferred to another product: In order to increase the amount of protein in soy beans, a gene from the Brazil nut was injected into the genome of the soy bean. In further investigations scientists proved that these so-called transgenetic soy beans could cause allergic reactions in people allergic to nuts. The production of transgenetic soy beans was then immediately stopped. In this case the food industry reacted with a measure of responsibility.

All genetically modified foodstuffs should be critically studied in this regard. We should not be confronted with reactions like the one that I heard about at a congress of a patient reacting to a tomato although he was "only" allergic to nuts. As it turned out, the tomato had been genetically revamped with a hazel nut gene, which explains the man's allergic reaction. One can only hope that this case report will someday be publicized more extensively in some well-known journal. One congress participant voiced the hope that we won't have to use a nutcracker to eat tomatoes in the future. But, then again, maybe genetic engineering will someday also be able to eliminate allergies. Everything has two sides to it.

Pro and contra genetic engineering

Manipulating the genetic makeup of foodstuffs is done in order to make the plants more resistant to insects, viruses, fungi, herbicides, or bacteria – and to increase the nutritional value of the product. Thus, genetic engineering strives to reduce the amount of pesticides needed. To date, the only plants that have been genetically manipulated are the soy bean and corn, with the goal of positively changing the nutritional characteristics, for example, to reduce the amount of cholesterol present.

With rice scientists tried to reduce the allergenicity via genetic engineering, but the result never came to market. Then they tried to suppress the protein that causes allergic reactions, but the process wasn't completely successful. The production of such hypoallergenic foods may not be feasible because of the many different allergens present that would have to be manipulated – and of course because of the great liability the producer would have to shoulder.

But do we really need to genetically fiddle with foods just to lower the amount of pesticides used? I don't think so.

Allergies and perfume

Everyone wants to smell good and float around in a cloud of fragrance. For a good few years now, this is no longer the sole province of women; scented body lotions, aftershaves and shower gels designed for and purchased by men (I prefer "Boss #1," a classic fragrance, which my wife also likes), bring some equality into this branch of our consumer society. As the perfume industry rubs its hands with glee, more and more people begin to itch. Perfume contains a variety of substances like rose oil, musk and sandalwood – all of which are potential allergens capable of producing red spots in the face, swelling, blistering and itching. So, if that's the case, grab your bottle of perfume and go see a doctor, and have him or her perform the various tests necessary to identify the allergen. Your doctor can also contact the manufacturer to get an idea of the individual substances to be tested, for early identification of the culprit. It may mean switching from Chanel No. 5 to Charlie – quite a change I admit! To end on a sensitive macho note: Success is a man's best perfume. But, men, if you agree with that, be careful of smelling like Al Bundy at his best.

Nail polish can also cause allergic reactions, whereby the source is usually the solvent used. Switch to another polish with a different solvent. There are numerous alternatives available.

Exotic allergens

The list of exotic allergens, that is to say rare ones, could be endless. I wish to mention just a few, some of which in the meantime have become important and are no longer rare, like storage mite and latex. I have already discussed exotic allergens like the red spider mite, spindle wood, *Ficus benjamina*, henna and gelatine, but most exotic allergens are job-related, such as peppermint leaves (for chemists), rubber gloves (for doctors and nurses), and unroasted coffee (for coffee manufacturers and dock workers).

A patient was tested with various house dust extracts over the course of several years without coming up positive. At the time he entered university to study biology, he was still suffering from unknown allergies. After casually mentioning to his doctor that his wardrobe was full of tiny beetles, he took some in to be tested. The manufactured extract tested positive, indicating that he was allergic to the beetles. Here we see that even the most insignificant observation can lead to the discovery of allergens.

Another rare allergy which can seriously interfere with one's enjoyment of life is a sperm allergy, when women show an allergic reaction to their partner's sperm.

In one known case a woman did actually develop an allergy to sperm after working as a lab assistant doing chemical tests in a doctor's office and a laboratory. Since she wants to have children of her own, she is now considering hyposensitization with a specific sperm extract. I will keep you up to date in the next editions on how her case is progressing. I'm curious myself.

Only a few reports describe successful cases of hyposensitization with sperm extract. The best protection – not only against AIDS – is of course a condom, as long as the partners are not allergic to latex. Luckily, a simultaneous allergy to rubber and sperm is extremely rare and has not yet been documented in literature on the subject.

We have only touched on the many exotic allergies out there – and new ones are being discovered daily that someday may in fact be important allergens for a greater number of people. One of the most important allergens will most likely be *Ficus benjamina*. By the time this edition appears, it is my opinion that the once exotic *Ficus* has evolved in to a full-blown allergen.

Allergens in the home – good luck, Sherlock!

Quite often you are required to have the skills of a Sherlock Holmes to be able to find and determine what causes allergies.

A friend of mine greeted her brother-in-law, who responded with an embrace. At dinner shortly afterwards she began constantly scratching her cheek. When she looked at her face in the bathroom mirror, she noticed a rash of tiny spots on her right cheek. When she asked her brother-in-law if he had recently switched aftershave he said no, but that he had just been to the vet with his dog, which he had carried on his arm. Since my friend worked for an allergologist and knew that she was allergic to dog hair, she realized that in greeting her brother-in-law she had come into contact with some dog hairs on his jacket. When these dog hairs rubbed against her cheek they caused the rash. If you wish, this was an "accidental" rub test (see p. 85). Thanks to her "allergological background," my friend was able to pinpoint her allergic response immediately, something an amateur could have had more trouble with.

Can animals also have allergies?

Like humans, animals can also react with allergies to certain substances. And as in humans, allergies in animals are on the increase. To date, allergies are known in dogs, cats and some horses (SÆTA, the Icelandic pony of Mrs. V. S.). Germany has a total of about 5 million pet dogs, and it has been estimated that some 10% suffer from allergies. The percentage in horses is not known, but they too can in any case become allergic.

An increasing number of horses (as well as a good number of human spectators, including myself) are reacting especially negatively to any military riding competition. Just remember the pictures from the Sydney Olympics in 2000.

Horses tend to react to dust from hay and straw, which could be in effect an allergic reaction to the mites present. The respiratory system is usually affected. But the skin can also react to insect bites (summer eczema, presumably caused by the saliva of the mosquito). Respiratory allergic reactions may also be found in dogs and cats, which are also prone to skin reactions, leading to urticaria, itching, reddening of the skin, ear and eye infections, or even loss of hair. The latter can be traced back to a licking dermatitis caused by increased licking by a dog or cat when the skin itches. Allergies are usually found in pedigree animals such as Golden Retriever, West Highland Terrier, Boxer and German Shepherd. Your normal stray hybrids have it easier: Because they have not been so strictly bred, they are not as prone to allergic diseases. And what does this tell us about the human race? Within animal breeds allergies are in any case passed on.

As in humans, an animal allergy can be diagnosed and treated. **This should always be done by a veterinarian.** Testing is done intracutaneously (see p. 86) with the respective allergenic extracts, adjusted to a different concentration than in humans. In dogs, for example, the animal has first to be sedated and the test spot shaved before testing begins. If, based on the anamnesis, the results of the skin test, and the *in vitro* tests, a therapy is considered advantageous, the concentration is a different one than in humans. Immunotherapy is usually done via subcutaneous injection. But just try to treat a cat and you'll experience its relationship to the tiger (see Fig. 22)! In such cases one should consider oral hyposensitization instead by

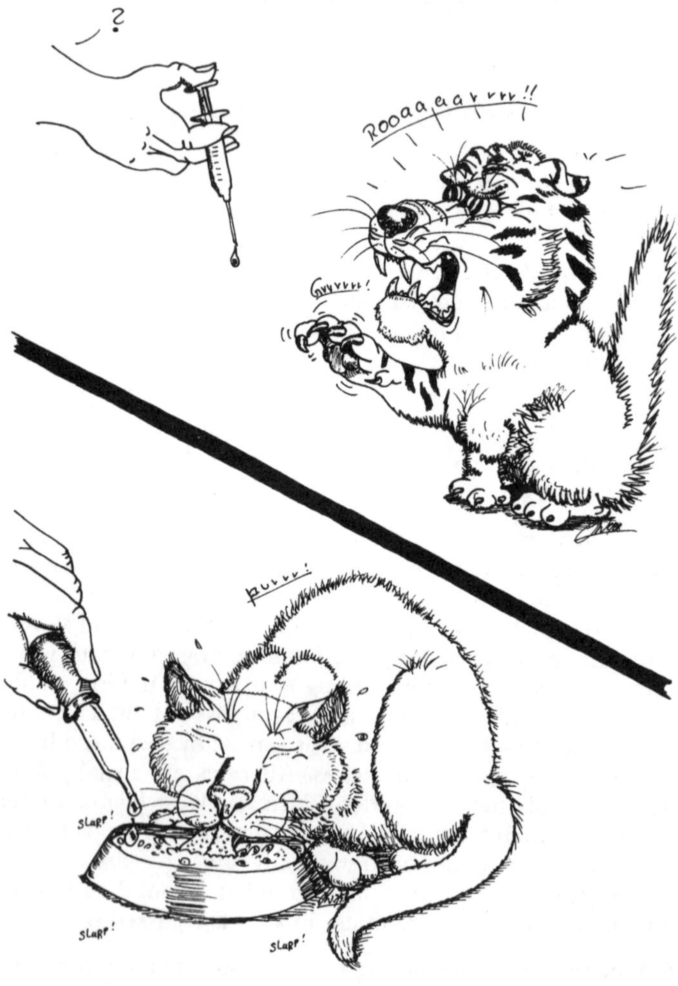

Figure 22. The "tiger-cat" – or: is gentle immunotherapy a real alternative? Clinical studies may someday tell.

giving the cat the respective allergen extract with its normal meals. Whether this is a good and productive method is another thing: There are to date no studies on this. It is also unclear exactly how long such a therapy should last – the times given vary between 3 months and forever.

The most successful immunotherapy in animals has been that with mites. In dogs with house dust mite allergy *Dermatophagoides farinae* is much more important than *Dermatophagoides pteronyssinus*. In humans the difference is not so great, and the two mites are responsible for similar numbers of problems. We desperately need more clinical studies concerning the length of therapy and its chance of success.

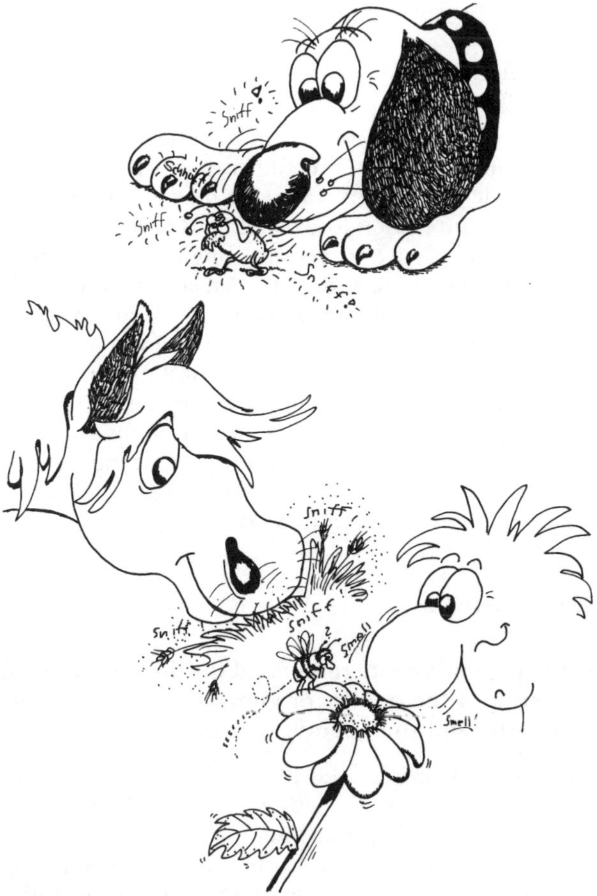

Figure 23. The sniff, snoop, and smell stages.

The most important sources of allergen are house dust mites and storage mites. They may be found not only in house dust, but in dry food as well. Dogs allergic to mites should thus be switched from dry to canned (wet) foods or home-cooked meals. Pollen as well can cause some allergic reactions in animals which can be treated. There have even been cases of dogs being allergic to cat hairs, for which immunotherapy has been successfully employed. The problem of allergic reactions in general is clearly growing, and research in animal allergies is still very much in its infancy. Here much research is demanded of veterinarians. The animals and of course their owners would be thankful for these efforts – animals are in fact often more thankful than humans. Simply put: Allergy can occur in the sniff, snoop, and smell stages (Fig. 23).

Choosing a doctor

It is possible in some cases for allergy sufferers themselves to locate the source of their allergies, but the various diagnostic tests which more precisely determine the allergens have to be carried out by a doctor. The question is therefore, what kind of doctor should you go to? If, at a specific place and certain time of day, your eyes always water, your nose always runs, or you even suffer asthma attacks, the person to see is an allergologist. However, ENT and lung specialists, pediatricians, dermatologists, and sometimes even internists include allergology in their expertise. You must describe your symptoms carefully, noting exactly when the symptoms occur, e. g., following a particular meal. You should also tell the doctor about any other allergy sufferers in the family (see p. 54). After questioning the patient, the doctor will perform a variety of *in vivo* and possibly also *in vitro* tests with allergen extracts, allergen disks or allergen test sticks.

Allergen extracts

Not only the patient's cooperation and the doctor's experience and expertise, but also the quality of allergenic extracts largely determines diagnostic and therapeutic success.

Today, many raw materials used in making allergen extracts are industrially manufactured and strictly controlled. House dust mites, for instance, are bred on a special medium from which they can be isolated and used – in their pure form – for manufacturing allergen extracts. Before they are made into extracts, all raw materials undergo testing (also under a microscope) to determine their purity. They are only used as extracts if they meet with the regulations set by the allergen extract manufacturers. Allergens, luckily, are water soluble proteins which can be manufactured through aqueous extraction. Using a variety of protein-chemical and immunobiochemical methods, the allergen composition and the activity of such extracts are then characterized and standardized. Since these methods are very specialized and in part extremely complicated, I shall not elaborate further at this point and risk boring you with a technical superstructure, although scientists find these methods very fascinating and exciting. If you are at all interested, I would be happy to supply you with the relevant literature on the characterization and standardization of allergen extracts. (Please enclose an envelope with the appropriate postage.)

In conclusion, I would like to stress that (contrary to what is sometimes claimed) allergen extracts *are* manufactured from selected raw materials and are carefully characterized and standardized using a variety of methods in order to provide doctors and patients with safe preparations and aid successful diagnosis and therapy.

What do all the numbers mean?

Numbers, numbers, numbers wherever you look, even on the allergen bottles. But every figure is significant, just like in your bank account (where I prefer the ones indicating that I'm in the black). Prick test bottles and therapy solution bottles carry labels containing many numbers: the name of the extract, the code number, storage conditions and the concentration, and lot numbers. The lot number enables the manufacturer to tell at a glance where and how the extract was manufactured. This is important in the event that a complaint is filed. The manufacturer keeps a so-called backup of every preparation in order to be able to quickly check the lot number if there is a complaint.

Storage

The preparations have to be stored as prescribed by the manufacturer and printed on the bottle. Therapy solutions from the pharmacy, for instance, shouldn't be transported for hours on the backseat of your car in the sun, but should be stored at 4–6°C (39–43°F) in the fridge. Therapy solutions should also not be frozen, as this destroys the allergenic activity. So don't store your allergen solutions in the deep freeze compartment, either. If the expiration date has passed, the preparation may no longer be used. The manufacturer only guarantees absolute quality up until the expiration date.

That was a short lesson on allergen extracts, not entirely irrelevant, in my opinion.

What are diagnostic and therapeutic extracts?

In vivo diagnosis: Allergic disorders are diagnosed via skin prick tests, intracutaneous tests, conjunctival test and provocation tests. These tests investigate the composition of allergen extracts.

The skin prick test

The first test the doctor will carry out is the (relatively painless) skin prick test. In this test, various drops of allergen solutions such as house dust mite, grass pollen, or cat epithelia are applied to the underside of a patient's arm, and the skin in the center of the drop is lightly pricked with a needle (see Fig. 24).

A prick test solution of house dust mites consists of an aqueous allergen extract of house dust mites, preserved with 0.2–0.5% phenol and 50% glycerin. Glycerin increases the stability of the extract and makes the drop stay on your arm without rolling off. If you are allergic to house dust mites, for instance, your skin will turn red, begin to itch, and break out in wheals within 15 minutes. As a result of pricking the upper layer of skin, the allergen reacts with the 5,000–10,000 heparinocytes occurring per mm^2 and located primarily near the capillaries. The histamine released typically causes the wheals and appearance of a rash. By measuring the diameter of the wheals, a doctor can approximately tell the degree of sensitization. As a comparison to the test with the allergen extract, a histamine positive solution (0.1 or 1%) is tested alongside the extract, and as a negative control a physiological saline solution is also often used. Histamine is used because it is released by the mast cell when it comes into contact with an allergen, and a pure histamine solution also causes a skin reaction.

By comparing the wheals caused by the allergen with those caused by the positive histamine test, a doctor can determine the degree of sensitization. The physiological saline solution (0.9% NaCl, sodium chloride) should not cause a wheal, and if it does, this is due to the mechanical stimulus. Thus the wheals caused by the allergen extract solution cannot really be assessed as positive, and in order to be

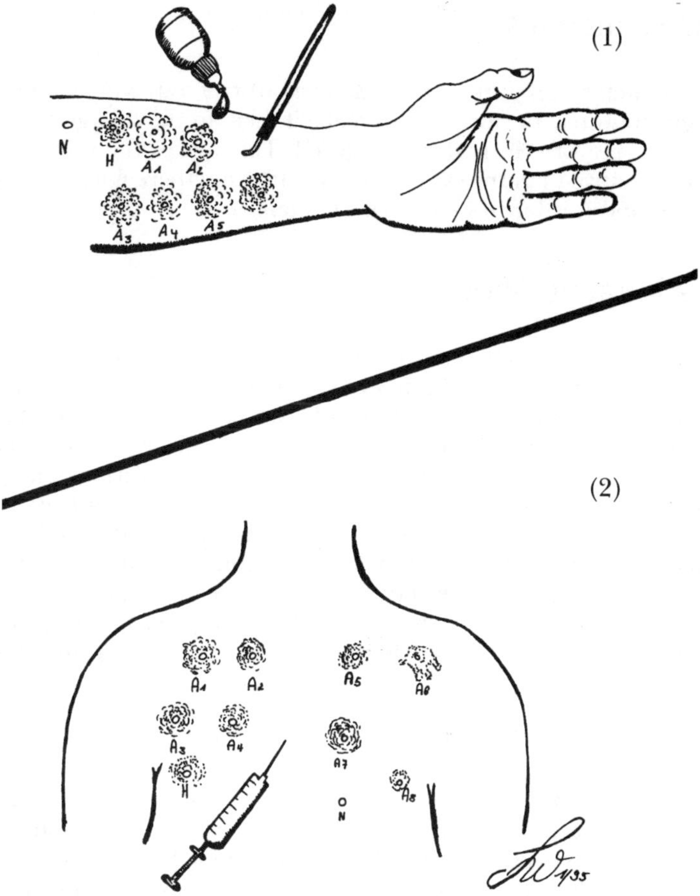

Figure 24. Skin prick test (1), A: allergen extract, H: positive histamine control, N: negative control (physiological saline solution); IC test (2).

certain about the allergy, another *in vitro* or *in vivo* test must be carried out.

The rub test

Due to its low sensitivity, the rub test is no longer commonly carried out. It can be particularly useful when a high degree of sensitization is suspected. The fur, animal hair, or food (such as a piece of apple) is rubbed on the inside of the patient's arm. A rash indicates a positive reaction caused by the release of histamine from the mast cells.

The scratch test

The scratch test is a more extreme form of rub test, and again is no longer routinely performed. To make it take up the allergen better, a larger area of skin is slightly injured. This makes the scratch test more sensitive than the skin prick test, although there is a risk of side effects, and it is far more difficult to control.

The intracutaneous test

The intracutaneous (IC) test is another form of skin test. The IC test solution often consists of a freeze dried allergen extract (similar to instant coffee powder) which is dissolved in an aqueous solution containing no glycerin, as this would cause a burning sensation where the extract is injected into the skin (see Fig. 24). Various allergen extracts are injected into the patient's back. This test is at least 1000 times more sensitive than the skin prick test. Compared with the skin prick test solution, the allergen concentration in the IC test solution is around 1000 times lower. The IC test is also a little bit more painful. Here too, by comparing the rash with that caused by the positive histamine test, a doctor can determine the degree of sensitization.

Limits to skin testing

The results of a skin test are largely dependent on the quality of the allergen extract, which should be clearly defined and standardized. As the wheal is caused by the release of histamine from the mast cells, skin tests only make sense after a patient has stopped using antihistamine drugs for 2–3 weeks. Antihistamine drugs strongly inhibit the release of histamine. If a patient has a skin disease it is also impossible to perform a skin test, and an *in vitro* test must be substituted.

Clinical research has shown that positive skin test results decrease the older the patient gets.

What other tests can determine allergies? The provocation test

Although only one or two allergens can be tested each day (albeit in increasing concentrations), the provocation test for determining allergies is still extremely useful. The provocation test consists of bron-

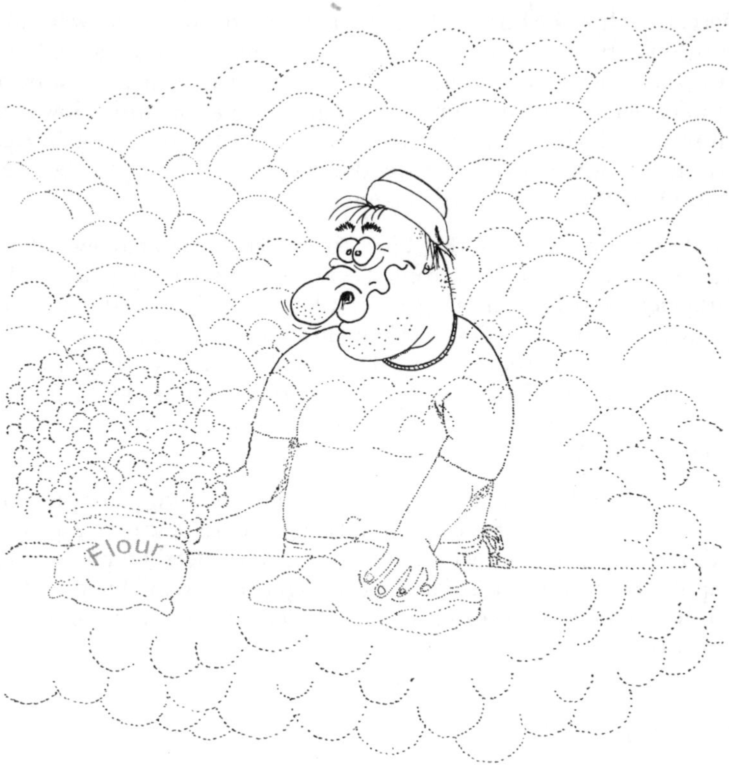

Figure 25. There's nothing like being provoked at work!

chial, nasal, conjunctival, and oral provocation. In the bronchial provocation test, patients inhale the allergen in different concentrations as an aerosol while their airway resistance is measured. This reading provides the doctor with information about the patient's general reaction.

In the nasal provocation test, different concentrations of the allergen extract are dribbled into the patient's nose. If the patient is allergic to the allergen, his or her nose may begin to run or he/she may start to sneeze, depending on the response typical of a particular disease such as hayfever.

In the conjunctival provocation test the allergen is applied – in the form of eyedrops – to the eye. Red and streaming eyes indicate a positive response.

The oral provocation test plays a major role in the diagnosis of food allergies. The patient swallows capsules consisting of a freeze dried allergen such as shrimp. If the patient is allergic, he or she will show a response typical of food allergies: discomfort, diarrhea, asthma, urticaria. This test is also performed with various concentrations of the allergen to ensure accuracy, beginning obviously with a low concentration which is gradually increased. In order to be certain that a given reaction is really positive, the patient is given a placebo, i. e., a capsule without any allergen content.

Another provocation test (Fig. 25) is the workplace-related one, where the patient is directly confronted with the allergens just as in the workplace. A baker suffering from allergies (baker's asthma is primarily an allergic reaction to flour dust) is instructed to work with flour in one of the rooms at the doctor's office. If allergic symptoms arise, the source of the allergy can be identified as the flour, the enzyme α-amylase (one of its constituents) or even ricemeal bugs, known to be in flour.

To save themselves the time-consuming and not altogether pleasant *in vivo* tests, allergy sufferers should keep a record of their symptoms, jotting down when and where they occur. Your detailed notes could simplify the doctor's task of making a diagnosis, and might even spare you the inconvenience of some of the tests, save the short confirmation checks.

In vitro methods

If you are dead set against undergoing *in vivo* tests, it is possible to have your allergies tested using *in vitro* methods. Serum from your body is needed for these tests. It is obtained from your blood through centrifugation, which separates the serum from the blood cells. Six ml of blood yields 2–3 ml of serum, and 1 ml of serum is all that is required for testing 20 different allergens. This test can be carried out irrespective of whether the patient is taking antihistamine drugs or suffers from a skin disease, factors which often render a skin prick test impossible, and at best impede the results significantly.

If a patient displays a high degree of sensitivity to an allergen, to the point that it is suspected that skin tests may trigger too extreme a response, *in vivo* tests should certainly be replaced by *in vitro* tests. The only *in vivo* test which could still be safely performed with a highly sensitized patient would be a rub test.

What are the *in vitro* tests and what do they do? They are called RIA (analysis of specific IgE by radio-immuno-assay), RAST or ELISA (enzyme-linked immuno-sorbent assay) or EAST. Figure 26 simply

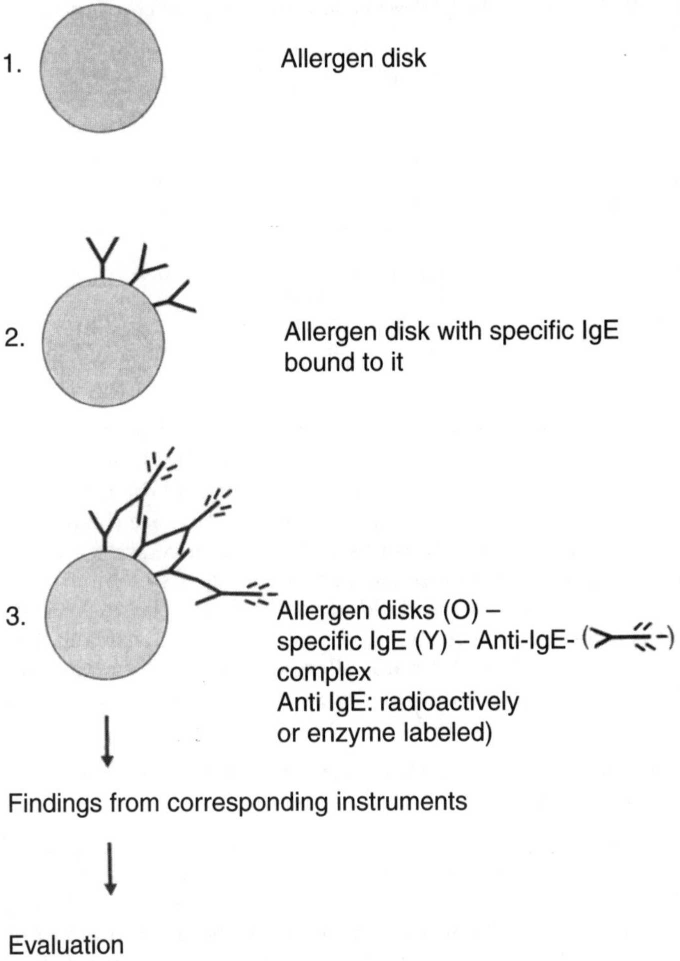

Figure 26. RAST or EAST. 1, allergen disk; 2, specific IgE binds to the allergen disk; 3, radioactive or enzyme labeled anti-IgE binds to the specific IgE. The higher the content of specific IgE in the serum, the more will bind to the allergen disk, and the more anti-IgE will bind to the specific IgE.

and briefly illustrates this method of testing. The patient's serum is applied to a paper disk, to which the allergen is chemically bound. The specific IgE (house dust mite, for example) present in the serum of a person allergic to the critters, binds with the allergen on the paper, which is washed to remove any unbound substances. It is then incubated with enzyme or radioactively labeled anti-IgE. The labeled

Table 1. Analysis of specific IgE level in different allergy sufferers, established via the RAST classes.

Sera	Allergen disks	RAST classes
Reference		
Reference A	Reference	4
Reference B	Reference	3
Reference C	Reference	2
Reference D	Reference	1
Test		
Patient 1	Cat epithelia	3.3
Patient 2	House dust mite	4.2
Patient 3	Birch pollen	1.1
Patient 4	Grass pollen	0.8

anti-IgE binds to the specific IgE on the allergen disk. The more the specific IgE binds to the disk, the more the anti-IgE binds, the higher the level of specific IgE in the patient's serum, and the more strongly he is likely to be sensitized to the allergen, in this case the house dust mite. By comparing the findings with a reference system based on different IgE concentrations of sera (mostly grass or birch), the degree of sensitization can be divided into different classes. Usually the classification ranges from 0 – 4 (4 = very strong, 3 = strong, 2 = not so strong, 1 = weak and 0 = not allergic). Table 1 shows an analysis of the specific IgE content in the sera of patients allergic to cats, house dust mite, birch, and grass pollen.

The allergenic class for each allergy sufferer is always based on the reference system.

If you want to screen for allergies, you can use an allergen disk to which several allergens have been bound, e. g., a mixture of animal epithelia like cat, dog, horse, guinea pig and hamster. In the case of a positive reaction, the individual disks can be used to pinpoint the culprit. The advantage to be had using the group allergen disk is that it covers several allergens at once, supplying a clear "yes" or "no."

A simple and easy method of proving the existence of an allergy on the basis of the specific IgE value is the allergen test strip. Different allergen fields as well as control fields (both positive and negative) are placed on a plastic strip (Fig. 27). The patient's serum is first put in a tube and the test strip left in the serum for a while and afterwards washed under running water. Then, the strip is put into a second fluid (conjugate), washed again, and finally put into a third fluid, the substrate. Now the strip is removed and read: If the patient is reacting to some allergen present on the strip (i.e., is sensitized to that allergen), then the respective field will turn blue. The

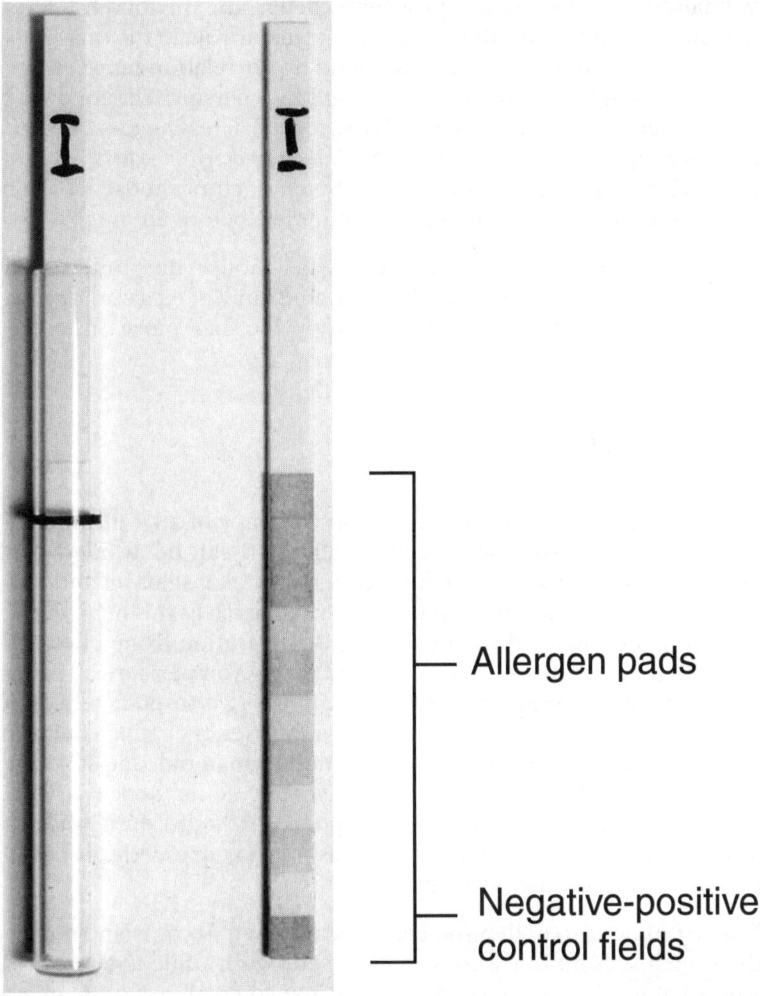

Figure 27. Allergen test strip with the allergen fields and the postive and negative control fields. The following allergens (among others) are available (from top to bottom): grass pollen, birch pollen, mugwort pollen, plantain pollen, dog hair, cat hair, *Alternaria tenuis* (mold), house dust mite, negative and positive control fields. *Left:* before testing; *right:* after testing with resulting coloring effect.

greater the sensitization, the more intensive the color. The coloring is compared to a standard card and the grade of sensitization is classified between 0 and 4. With this system one can handily classify human specific IgE.

By analyzing the serum, it is possible to determine the total IgE level in a patient, but the test does not play the major role in the diagnosis of allergic disorders. Studies have found no correlation between the total level of IgE and that of specific IgE in a person. The following is the recommended order in which to proceed in testing for allergies: *have your case history recorded by a doctor, then undergo skin tests, in vitro tests and, if necessary, provocation tests*. Some doctors choose, at their own discretion, to perform a provocation test before an *in vitro* test.

Now you've heard a lot about allergens, house dust mites and rock'n'roll, exotic allergens, IgE, histamine, and *in vivo* and *in vitro* tests, but nothing whatever about therapy. We shall move on to this now.

Avoiding allergens

Avoiding allergens altogether is the best therapy of all, but unfortunately not always so easy. But many allergens can be avoided. For people allergic to lobster, the implication is total abstention and having to "make do" with the mundane herring, harsh as this may sound. It is probably equally difficult to imagine separation from a beloved pet, which unfortunately doesn't stop at giving you pleasure but goes on to give you allergies as well. If you're allergic to penicillin, you have to switch to an alternative, if it's strawberries, try eating cherries, if it's latex you should wear gloves of another material, and if you're allergic to milk you should switch to hypoallergenic food. But what do you do if you have an allergy to pollen or house dust mites or insect poison? In summer, bees and wasps lurk impatiently, just waiting for an opportunity to sting!

If you're allergic to pollen you could escape to an Arctic island during the pollen season, but who would do your work while you're away? And what would your boss have to say? You could always get yourself a wonderful helmet with a pollen filter (Fig. 28), but you're unlikely to create a new fashion. In all likelihood you'll just start having social problems and your hairstyle will suffer. If you're allergic to house dust mites you could try emigrating to the north pole, not the kindest solution of all but you have my personal guarantee that there are no house dust mites there. As you can see, some of the possible methods of avoiding allergens are a little too radical, and not necessarily very practical. This is why there is the possibility for sufferers from pollen, house dust mites, insect poison, even animal hair and mold allergies to hyposensitize (desensitize) themselves with the help of a doctor.

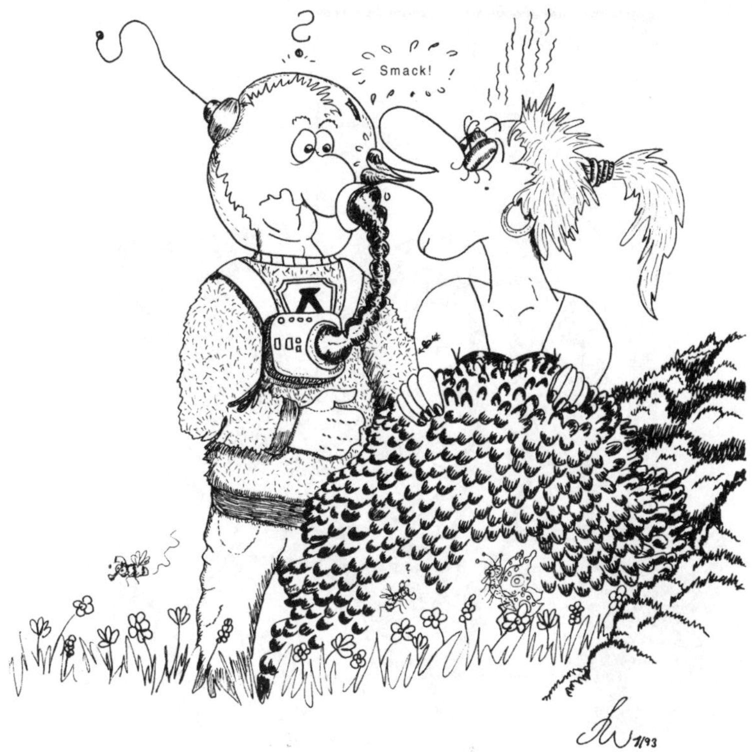

Figure 28. Somehow I just can't seem to get close to you! Smack!

Hyposensitization - desensitization

In Europe, hyposensitization is carried out in around 98% of cases by way of depot allergen preparations. Aqueous extracts are primarily used in therapy in the United States, while depot preparations are only used in 20% of cases. This may simply be for reasons of "tradition." In depot preparations, the allergen or allergoid (chemically modified allergen) is bound to a special carrier. The "depot" method means that the allergen or allergoid extract, administered via subcutaneous injection, is deposited little by little into the body and thus represents a safe and effect form of therapy, as well as protection against allergens.

Prerequisites for the success of hyposensitization are the patient's cooperation, the doctor's experience and expertise, and the quality of the allergen or allergoid extracts, which must be both characterized and standardized.

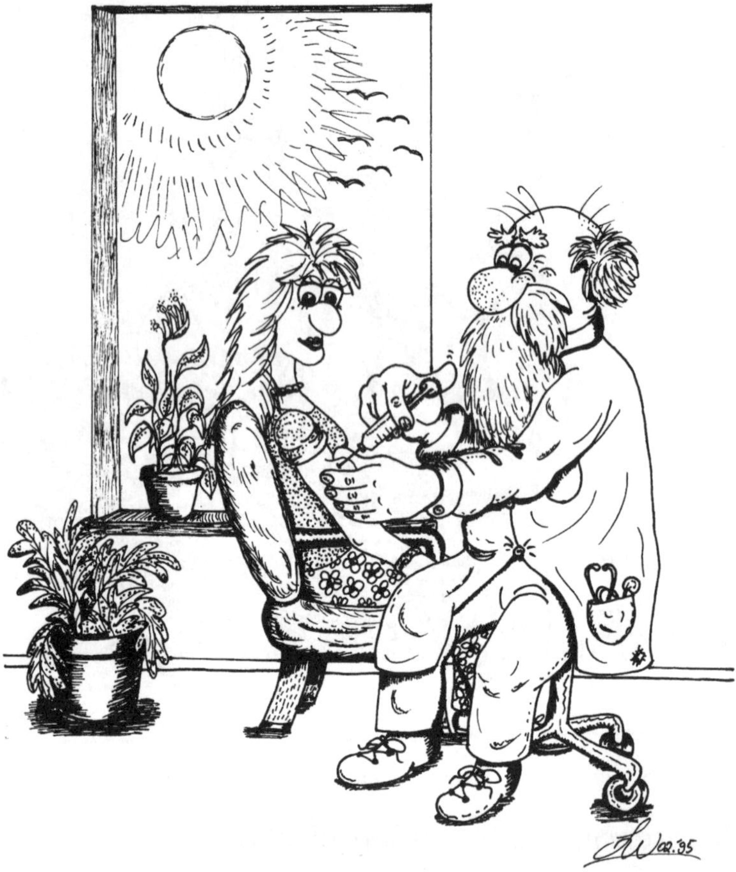

Figure 29. Hyposensitization. Make sure you follow your doctor's instructions.

What is hyposensitization? It is an (almost) painless procedure in which a patient is subcutaneously injected with various doses of an allergen or allergoid (see Fig. 29).

Therapy extracts only consist of the actual aggravating allergens, and the doses are always individual and cannot be administered schematically. Therapy usually takes place over a period of 2–3 years and, as a rule, is continued for an entire year after the symptoms have disappeared. Regarding house dust mite allergies, some people even suggest that therapy should be continued for life – perish the thought!

The success rate for people who are allergic to grass, tree, and herb pollen, as well as bees and wasps, lies around 90%, while for those allergic to house dust mites it is between 70 and 80%. Even people who are allergic to cats have a good chance of success, and to increase this chance, you are best off getting rid of your cat (or at least showering it once a week).

Initial clinical studies show that allergies to foodstuffs (e. g., apples) can be successfully treated via the cross-reactive, pollen-associated allergens (birch pollen). Although this method of immunotherapy is still in its infancy, it promises to be an interesting and fruitful field.

Immunologically speaking, hyposensitization allows IgG antibodies to be created which protect the patient from the allergen.

A high level of specific IgG, however, cannot be considered as evidence of clinical success. It is only a sign that the patient's immune system has been stimulated by the therapy. Unfortunately, there exist no serological tests which might indicate whether or not therapy has been successful. The best indication of success is when a patient is able to say: "I'm feeling a lot better, Doctor, my nose has stopped running and my asthma is gone." This is exactly what doctors love to hear, and what every patient would love to tell them.

How can you physically illustrate the success of hyposensitization? If a person is allergic to bees, he or she can be provoked directly. Under medical supervision, the patient is stung by a bee. If the therapy has been successful, nothing untoward happens. This method is obviously the most violent, but it does give the patient the necessary confidence to go outdoors and enjoy nature in the summer months. People suffering from house dust mites and pollen allergies can be checked by a bronchial provocation test. Therapy is proven to be effective when the resistance of patient's airways when confronted with the allergen is not as great as it was before therapy.

Desensitization – what must you look out for?

It is vital that the patient stay in the doctor's waiting room for half an hour (this depends on the respective recommendations of the country's different societies) after receiving the injection so that the doctor can swiftly administer the necessary first aid if there are any side effects. Additionally, patients should take care to avoid physical exertion for several hours after therapy and so avoid putting any strain on the cardiovascular system. Further points to be observed are listed at the back of the book.

If a patient prefers not to undergo a series of shots, he or she can try oral or sublingual therapy. The patient swallows the allergens in liquid form for the oral therapy, and in sublingual therapy holds the liquid mixture under his or her tongue for several minutes before spitting it out. In this therapy as well, the allergen is administered in various doses, starting at a very low concentration and increasing bit by bit before reaching the final concentration, the "maintenance dose." In contrast to classical therapy, as yet there are no reliable figures confirming the effectiveness of these types of therapy. They appear to enjoy more success with young children than adults, and certainly provide an alternative.

Non-causal therapy

Instead of undergoing causal therapy such as hyposensitization, patients also have the option of non-causal therapy in which they are treated with medication such as cortisone. Unlike hyposensitization, which takes place over a period of 3 years, such forms of therapy must be continued for the patient's entire life. As an alternative to hyposensitization, cortisone therapy must be under the strict observation of a doctor, as long-term administration of cortisone can produce side effects. Cortisone therapy has fewer side effects when topical cortisone preparations are used. The cortisone is sprayed directly into the nose to reach the mucous membranes or directly to the lungs via aerosol.

Hyposensitization can also cause side effects, of course, as can be said for virtually all forms of medication. Some scientists and doctors even go so far as to claim that a medicament without side effects cannot be effective. Whether or not this is true must be left open.

Postscript 1

Because the range of existing allergies is extremely large, it is impossible to cover all types of allergies in a book such as this. This book is simply intended as an introduction to the subject. There are a multitude of other books on the market addressing the problem of allergies far more intensively than I am willing or able. Although there are also other types of allergies, my primary goal was to discuss the early reaction types, i. e., allergies that are mediated by IgE, as they are my specific field.

In conclusion, I would like to mention one final allergy from which nearly everyone suffers: Gninromyadnom allergy (a little backward thinking is called for here, although otherwise I hope you are generally positive and forward thinking). I would suggest the following

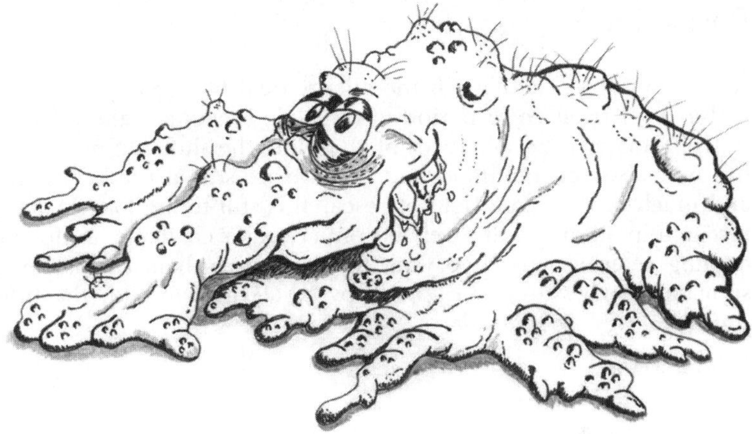

Figure 30. How an allergy might look – squish, squash.

therapy: lie still and wait for Tuesday, request vacation, or simply keep sleeping.

In Figure 30 you see how my niece, the illustrator, pictures an allergy in her worst nightmares. What do you think allergies look like?

That's it.

Postscript 2

Around 15–20% of the American population (as well as nearly 30% of the German population and 20–40% of the population of the UK) suffers from allergies, and the number is increasing all the time with more and more young people being affected. The number of asthma victims is nearly equal to that of traffic casualties. And although we know far more than we did 20 years ago about what allergenic materials contain and what causes allergic reactions, there is still a wide area open for study. We have excellent asthma clinics, institutes, doctor's offices, doctors, professors and scientists researching in the field and treating allergy patients. Nonetheless, it is my opinion that we should build allergy research centers where specialists from a variety of countries and a variety of fields such as medicine, chemistry, biology, immunology and computer science could *cooperate* in their study of allergies in order to disempower allergies, the hostages of humanity. The ultimate goal is for medical and scientific professionals alike to be able to say: "Allergy Made Simple."

Postscript 4

As clearly shown, activity in the allergy field has greatly increased within a relatively short period of time. No longer are allergic reactions in humans the sole focus of attention, the situation in animals has now also become important. But we are still at the beginning, and much of this large field of research is still to be done. Allergy research in animals will surely become a major challenge to up and coming veterinarians, who want to distinguish themselves. Maybe someday a new work will appear by a veterinarian with the title: *Animal Allergy Made Simple.*

Who knows?

Postscript 5

You think you've said everything that needed to be said – and then something new happens that just has to be included in the new edition. I find particularly exciting the studies conducted on the allergenicity of parasites in foodstuffs and the country/city phenomenon "Back to Nature." But is that really all that new? Certainly not: The great French philosopher Jean-Jacques Rousseau is said to harbored such thoughts back in 1750 (without really saying the words "Back to Nature"). He was of the opinion that the human being, after once being born, was continually being corrupted from that natural, primeval state by societal pressures and science. Thus, he did not mean it as it is often (erroneously) employed in the discussion on allergies. We shall see whether the country/city discussion will continue to play a major role or whether it is a flash in the allergological pan. The discussion will surely not last a long as those surrounding the philosophical musings of Rousseau.

We shall see.

Tips for allergy sufferers

1. Avoid anything that irritates the airways such as cigarette smoke.
2. Keep your living area, especially your bedroom, free of dust. We recommend buying furniture and carpeting which can be wiped clean.
3. Don't keep any pets.
4. Discuss all career plans with your allergologist.
5. Avoid exposing yourself to allergens when you have the 'flu.
6. Depending on where you live, try to keep your windows shut at certain times of day or year when pollen is in the air.
7. Wash your hair daily when airborne pollen is doing the rounds.
8. If you're allergic to insect poison, always carry for example an auto- injector.
9. If you're allergic to latex, wear a necklace or bracelet to let people know.
10. Keep a record of your symptoms and write everything down, regardless of how unimportant it may seem.

Preventative measures for the bedroom if you suffer from house dust mite allergy

1. Have your own personal bedroom, to be used for no activity other than sleeping.
2. Animals and cigarette smoke should be forbidden entry to the bedroom.
3. Use only the following floor coverings: linoleum, wood, stone or cork, as they are easy to clean.
4. Avoid objects which collect dust.
5. Use simple furniture and washable curtains

6. Replace your old mattress with a new one covered with special, mite-proof material.
7. Replace old quilts and eiderdown bedding and cover with mite-proof covers.
8. Wash your bedding regularly.

How to reduce the risk of insect bites

1. Be extra careful in the summer and when participating in outdoor activities.
2. Watch what you eat outside: Avoid jam, honey, sweet fruits, and soft drinks.
3. Always wear long pants and shoes on grass or when walking through fields. Wear gloves when gardening.
4. Avoid wearing light colored clothing. Perfume, scented soaps, and hairspray attract insects.
5. Remove all nests and sticks near the house. (Don't do it yourself if you're an allergy sufferer.)
6. Stay away from insect feeding grounds such as potting compost, cloverfields, orchards of ripe fruits, and fruit and vegetable stands.
7. Always wear a necklace or bracelet which identifies you as being allergic.
8. Always carry an auto-injector or inhaler for emergencies.
9. Contact a doctor immediately after taking emergency measures.

Hyposensitization: Hints for allergy patients

1. Specific hyposensitization involves injections given at regular intervals. Be conscientious about keeping all appointments.
2. Stay at the doctor's for at least 30 minutes (see p. 95) after each injection, as the following allergic responses may occur:
   - Reddening, swelling and itching at the injection site
   - Runny, tickly nose
   - Itchy, streaming eyes
   - Shortness of breath, difficulty breathing, tickly feeling in the back of the throat
   - Itching and spotting of the skin, nettle rash
   - Weakness, weariness, discomfort
   - Itching of the palms of the hands and soles of the feet as well as the tongue

   If you notice one or more of these symptoms, report them to your doctor immediately. If they occur after you have left the doctor's office, contact him or her immediately.
3. Avoid physical activity for several hours after every injection.
4. Avoid drinking alcohol or eating sumptuous meals before and after every injection.
5. For the duration of the therapy, only take medication that has been prescribed by your doctor. Discuss with him or her any innoculations you might need.
6. While still in therapy, avoid or limit contact with the substances which cause your allergies.
7. Before every injection, tell your doctor how your body reacted to the last one.
8. If your state of health changes during therapy, report this to your doctor. Women must report if they are pregnant or if they become pregnant while in therapy.
9. Always let your doctor know in advance if you must leave the area where you are being treated (e.g., if you want to travel).
10. Discuss with your doctor when and where to travel in view of your allergies.

This may sound a little dangerous, but if you keep all the points in mind, most of the time nothing will happen.

Cross-reactive allergens

Cross-reactivity means that different substances produce the same allergens.

Allergens	*Cross-reactive allergens*
Pollen/pollen	
Birch	Alder, hazel, beech (red and hornbeam), ash (partial)
Poplar	Willow
Grasses such as *Phleum pratense*, etc.	Grains such as rye, barley, oats, wheat
Mugwort	Camomile, sometimes: ragweed, sunflower, daisy, *Euonymus europaea*
Lilac	Ash, olive tree
Mites	
House dust mite *Dermatophagoides pteronyssinus*	*Dermatophagoides farinae;* sometimes: red tree spider, storage mites *Acarus siro, Lipidoglyphus destructor, tyrophagus putrescentiae*
Blomia Tropicalis	Probably with *Blomia tjibodas, Blomia kulagini* (still under discussion)
Foodstuffs/foodstuffs	
Celery	Carrots, watermelon, cucumber
Flour (e.g., wheat)	Rye, oat and corn flour, rice, sesame seeds, poppy-seeds, rye grains (ground)
Molds	
Alternaria tenuis	Sometimes: *Stemphylium*
Candida	With other types of *Candida*
Pollen-associated cross-reactive foods	
Birch	Usually only partially: fresh pitted/stone fruits, fruits such as **apples** (especially Granny Smith, Golden Delicious), nuts especially hazel nuts, also in processed form (in chocolate bars, cookies, etc.), carrots, raw tomatoes, celery, kiwi

Grasses	Usually only partially: raw potatoes, soy bean, peanut, pea, kiwi
Mugwort	Herbs, **celery**, carrots, lychee, onions, camomile tea
Ragweed	Melon, camomile
Mites/foodstuffs	
Dermatophagoides pteronyssinus	Crustaceans, lobster, shrimp, crabs, pawn (usually only partially)
Feathers	
Bird feathers such as those from parakeets or canaries	Possibly chicken egg
Medicines	
Penicillin	Possibly Cephalosporin, Amoxicillin
Miscellaneous	
Latex (e.g., rubber gloves, condoms, balloons, etc.)	Banana, avocado, papaya, chestnut, kiwi, *Ficus benjamina*
Gelatin (e.g., in gummy bears, yogurt, etc.)	Blood volume expander, plasma expander
Cat hairs	Pork
Venison hairs (deer, stag)	Cow hairs
Kitchen cockroach *Blatella germanica*	Kitchen cockroach *Periplaneta americanica*

The allergenicity of fruits and vegetables

Fruits/Nuts

Apples

- Reactions vary according to type: Golden Delicious, Granny Smith, Jonagold, and Braeburn have a higher allergenic activity than Boskop, Jamba, or Gloster.
- The allergenic potency depends on the state of ripeness, i.e., allergenicity increases with ripeness.
- Heat destroys the allergen. Thus, apple jellies, cooked apples, apple juice, and apple pancakes are well suited.

Almonds

- Heat can reduce the allergenicity, depending on the part of the nut one reacts to.
- Reactions do not vary by type.

Hazel nuts

- Allergenicity not reduced by heat.
- Very potent allergen. Caution: even very small amounts can produce allergic reaction.
- Often hidden allergen especially in sweets, chocolate products, cookies.

Peanuts

- Allergenicity not reduced by heat or any other manufacturing processes
- Very potent allergen. Caution: even very small amounts can produce allergic reaction.
- Important hidden allergen, e.g., in pastries, sweets, chocolate products.
- The peanut is not really a nut, but a legume (like the soy bean).

Grains

- Heat may destroy the allergenicity, depending the part one reacts to.
- Cross-reactions between different types of grains occur. Often, however, only one or two types are clinically relevant.
- Unhusked grains have a higher allergenicity than processed grains.

Vegetables

Celery

- Heat may destroy the allergenicity, depending on the part one reacts to.
- Important hidden allergen often used as in seasonings and processed foods (instant meals and fast food).

Soy

- Heat may destroy the allergenicity, depending on the part one reacts to.
- Reactions do not vary by type.
- Important hidden allergen, e.g., in baked goods and pastries, sweets, meats, sports drinks and baby formula.
- Other legumes: Be careful with peanuts (see above). Only rarely are several other legumes (pea, bean, chickpea, lentil) simultaneously problematic.

Carrot

- Heat destroys the allergenicity. Thus, avoid eating raw carrots.

Potato

- Heat usually destroys the allergenicity, so that cooked potatoes are well tolerated.
- Reactions are usually contact eczemas or sneezing while peeling potatoes.

Herbs and Spices

Herbs

- Dried herbs are better tolerated than fresh ones.
- Reactions also to teas (e.g., camomile).

Spices

- Spices can withstand heat very well.
- Some spices are hidden allergens in foods when contents are not declared in detail (e.g., pepper, celery).

If you are atopic or react to pollen-associated allergens (see cross-reactivity), that doesn't mean that will automatically react to all "fruits." That may be case, but it need not be the case.

Table 2. Biogenetic amines in foodstuffs. During tests with native materials, biogenetic amines can create false positive reactions, e.g., during skin prick tests.

Development through enzymatic decarboxylation of amino acids (e.g., via microorganisms):	
Histamine (examples), in mg/kg:	
Spoiled fish	2000–5000
Sauerkraut	0–100
Tilsit cheese	ca. 37
Emmental cheese	0–2000
Salami	0–280
Yeast extract	up to 2000
Red wine	0–22 (mg/l)
White wine	1–5 (mg/l)
Tomatoes	20
Tyramine (examples), in mg/kg:	
Fish	0–500
Cheese	0–950
Bananas	7–11
Sauerkraut	20–95
Chocolate	0–25
Yeast extract	66–2260
Wine	0.4–3.6 (mg/l)
Tomatoes	4
Serotonin (5-hydroxytryptamine), in mg/kg:	
Bananas	23–78
Tomatoes	12

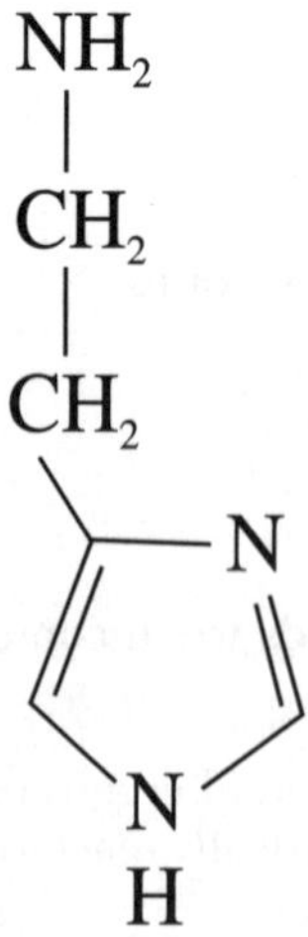

Figure 31. Histamine

Table 3. Physical characteristics of the major human immunoglobulin classes.

WHO name*	IgG	IgA	IgM	IgD	IgE
Molecular weight (Daltons)	150,000	160,000	900,000	185,000	200,000
Concentration in normal serum (mg/ml)	8–16	1.4–4	0.5–2	0–0.4	17-450**
% of total immuno-globulin	80	13	6	0–1	0.002
Carbohydrate content (%)	3	8	12	13	12

*WHO = World Health Organization; **in ng/ml

Index

AMERICAN ACADEMY OF ALLERGY & IMMUNOLOGY

611 E. Wells Street
Milwaukee, WI 53202
800-822-ASMA (2762)

United States Pollen Calendar

This state calendar is designed to depict the pollen seasons in the United States during average conditions. Local weather and individual sensitivity will determine the potential for allergic symptoms. The data shows general lengths of seasons, not taking into consideration pollen density. This information is not intended to replace physician advice. Contact your allergist if you have any questions.

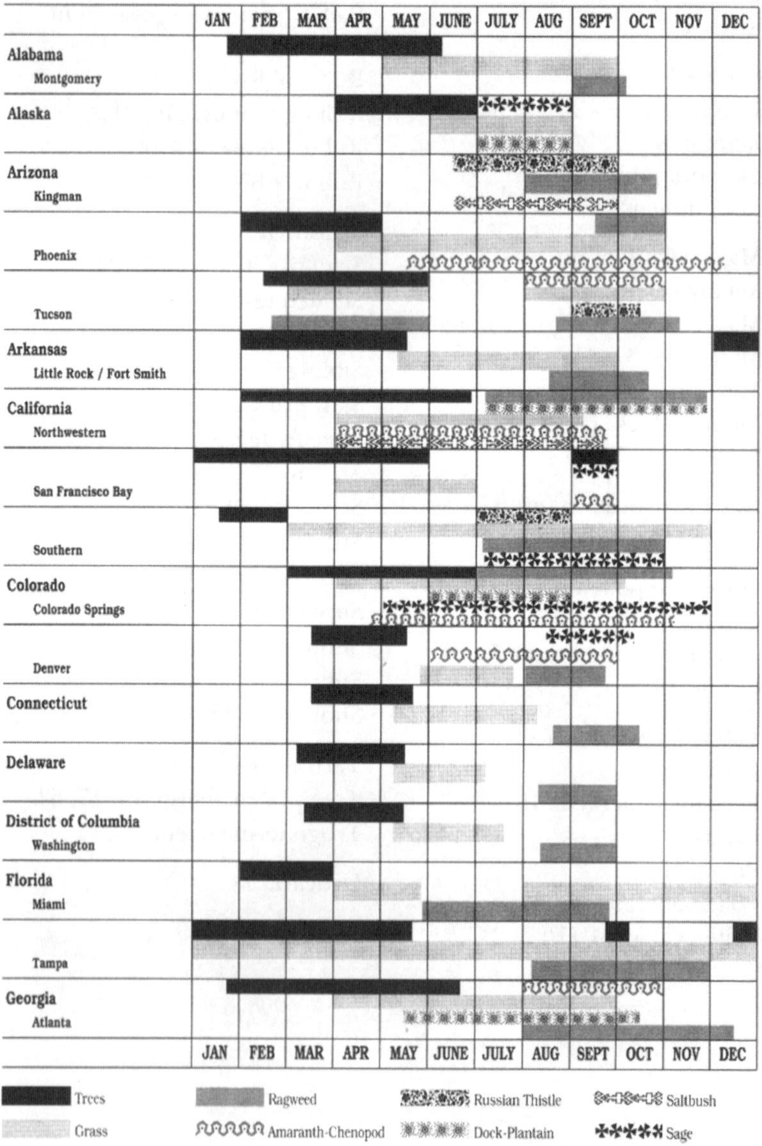

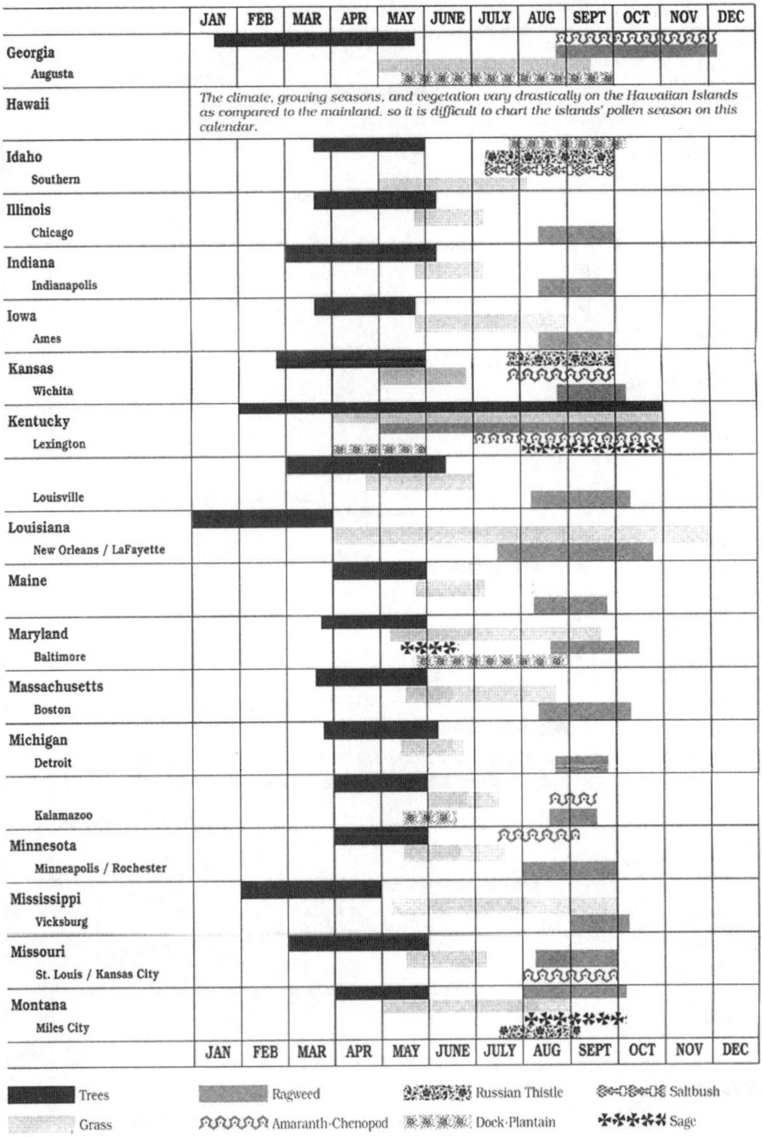
JAN FEB MAR APR MAY JUNE JULY AUG SEPT OCT NOV DEC
Georgia
Augusta
Hawaii
The climate, growing seasons, and vegetation vary drastically on the Hawaiian Islands as compared to the mainland, so it is difficult to chart the islands' pollen season on this calendar.
Idaho
Southern
Illinois
Chicago
Indiana
Indianapolis
Iowa
Ames
Kansas
Wichita
Kentucky
Lexington
Louisville
Louisiana
New Orleans / LaFayette
Maine
Maryland
Baltimore
Massachusetts
Boston
Michigan
Detroit
Kalamazoo
Minnesota
Minneapolis / Rochester
Mississippi
Vicksburg
Missouri
St. Louis / Kansas City
Montana
Miles City
JAN FEB MAR APR MAY JUNE JULY AUG SEPT OCT NOV DEC
Trees
Grass
Ragweed
Amaranth-Chenopod
Russian Thistle
Dock-Plantain
Saltbush
Sage

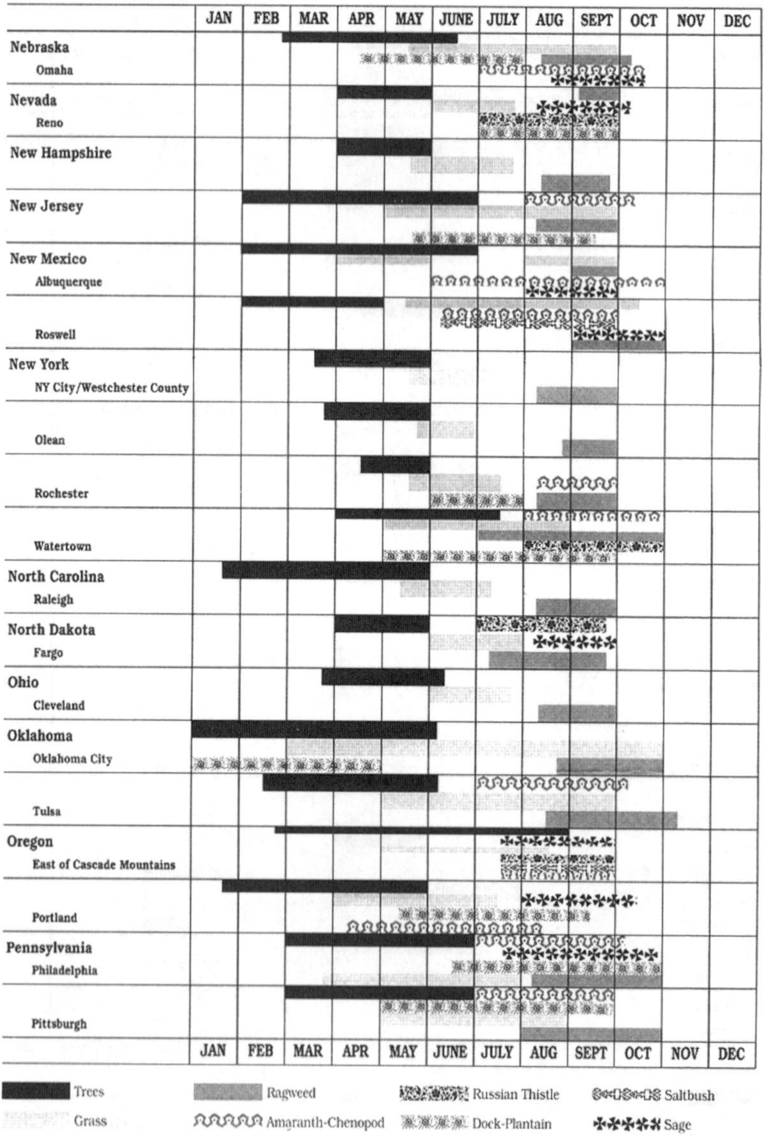
JAN FEB MAR APR MAY JUNE JULY AUG SEPT OCT NOV DEC
Nebraska
Omaha
Nevada
Reno
New Hampshire
New Jersey
New Mexico
Albuquerque
Roswell
New York
NY City/Westchester County
Olean
Rochester
Watertown
North Carolina
Raleigh
North Dakota
Fargo
Ohio
Cleveland
Oklahoma
Oklahoma City
Tulsa
Oregon
East of Cascade Mountains
Portland
Pennsylvania
Philadelphia
Pittsburgh
JAN FEB MAR APR MAY JUNE JULY AUG SEPT OCT NOV DEC
Trees
Ragweed
Russian Thistle
Saltbush
Grass
Amaranth-Chenopod
Dock-Plantain
Sage

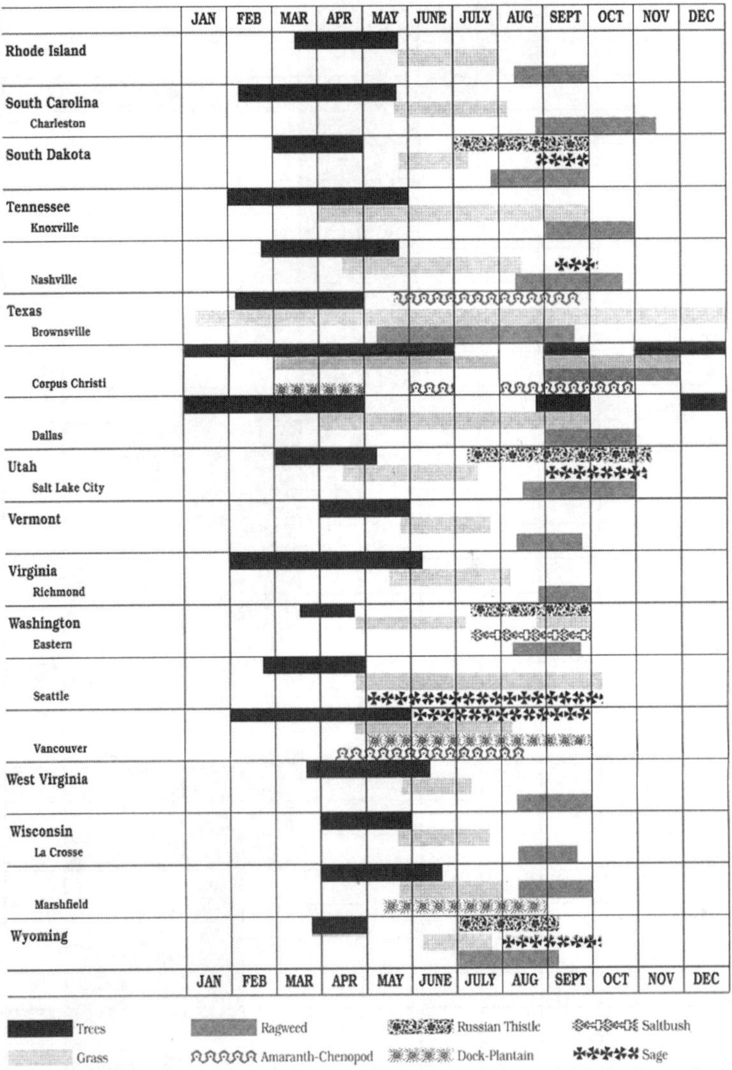

The US Pollen Calendar was reviewed by members of the American Academy of Allergy Asthma and Immunology's Aeroallergen Network, July 1993. All Aeroallergen Network members have been certified in pollen collection and identification.

5/95/10K

	January	February	March	April	May	June	July	August	September	October
Hazel	■	■	■	■						
Alder		■	■	■	■					
Elm		■	■	■	■					
Poplar		■	■	■						
Dandelion			■	■	■	■	■	■	■	■
Plantain				■	■					
Ash				■	■					
Beech				■	■					
Birch				■	■					
Oak				■	■	■				
Plane				■	■					
Sycamore				■	■	■				
Willow				■	■					
Meadow grass					■	■	■			
Yorkshire fog						■	■	■	■	
Rye grass						■	■	■		
Tall fescue						■	■			
Barley						■	■			
Rye						■	■	■	■	
Wheat						■	■	■	■	
Nettle						■	■	■		
Pellitory						■	■	■	■	■
Elder						■	■			
False acacia						■				
Chrysanthemum						■	■	■		
Marguerite (Daisy)						■	■	■		
Cocksfoot						■	■	■	■	
Timothy							■			
Maize							■	■		
Oats							■	■	■	
Mugwort							■	■	■	
Golden rod							■	■	■	
Aster								■	■	
Dahlia								■	■	■

Pollen calendar for realists (UK).